VIRGIN SEX

FOR GUYS

A NO-REGRETS GUIDE
TO SAFE AND HEALTHY SEX

Dr. Darcy Luadzers

Hatherleigh Press
New York • London

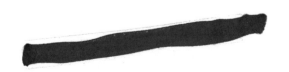

Hatherleigh Press
5-22 46th Avenue, Suite 200
Long Island City, NY 11101
www.hatherleighpress.com

CIP data available upon request.

ISBN-13: 978-1-57826-230-4
ISBN-10: 1-57826-230-5

Virgin Sex for Guys is available for bulk purchase, special promotions, and
premiums. For information on reselling and special purchase opportunities,
call 1-800-528-2550 and ask for the Special Sales Manager.

Interior design by Nancy Singer, and Deborah Miller
Cover design by Deborah Miller

10 9 8 7 6 5 4 3 2 1
Printed in Canada

Contents

Acknowledgments

Thank you to the many guys who gave me permission to share their very personal sexual stories. All of the guys were interviewed by me, some were referred by clients and friends, and others were asked by me to tell their stories. I felt like Dr. Alfred Kinsey, asking everyone he met to take their sexual history. In the movie *Kinsey*, about the first sex researcher (played by Liam Neeson), Dr. Kinsey, at times, looked kind of, well, strange or perverse, asking people he had never met, or anyone he met, about their sex life, including his own father! When I started my research to write this book, I started asking guys about their first time and relationships with girls, too. Surprisingly, I got lucky: the guys talked, and they were very kind, informative, and generous with their most personal and private stories of their lives. I found out that guys had a story to tell, too. They wanted other guys to know what they needed to know, to deal with girls and sex. Thank you to all the guys who saw beyond the weirdness in my asking them about their sex life, and focusing on what was important: giving guys a guide to safe and healthy sex.

Thank you to Jennifer DeChiara, my literary agent. Jennifer and I met at a Writer's Conference, where I gave her a 30 second pitch on the *Virgin Sex for Girls* book, on the way to an elevator. She kindly gave me her time, listened and said, "This is why I became an agent: to get this kind of book into the hands of teens." I thought I had died and gone to heaven. Here I was in New York City, among

25,000 other people at the Book Expo, trying to find someone to publish my book. I looked into Jennifer's eyes, saw that she understood my passion and purpose, and why I wrote *Virgin Sex for Girls*: to help teens. Period. Without my agent, this book for guys would have never happened. *Virgin Sex for Guys* is the result of her insight and personal vision.

Thank you to Andrea Au and Alyssa Smith at Hatherleigh Press, my editors. Thank you for your confidence in me and asking, "Why haven't you written a book for guys? We want a book for guys, too!" Books happen because publishers take a risk to spend their money on writers and topics they believe are important in the world. Thank you to Hatherleigh Press in believing not only in me, but realizing a guy's guide is essential for one half of the sexual equation.

Thanks to Maddie Wood, my teen editor, a high school junior at the Charleston County School of the Arts in South Carolina. Reviewing every word and page of the manuscript, part of Maddie's job was to make sure I didn't make any huge generation gap blunders in my writing. I am grateful for her help on the Sexual Dictionary and her kindness in not making fun of me when she pointed out an obvious (read: really stupid) awkward word or phrase. Maddie's best recommendation was that all her friends and any potential boyfriends must read Chapter Two, "Guys and Lies: How to Treat a Girl Right!"

Thanks to my husband, Dr. Jack Luadzers, who gave me a priceless gift in helping me write this book. Jack's a sex therapist, too, so he had the unique perspective of being both a therapist and a man, giving me a real guy's guidance on girls and sex. Jack and I spent hours and days talking about some of the ideas and topics in this book, discussing the different male and female views on subjects, from how to treat girls right, to date rape, and how to make a girl feel safe, sexually speaking. Thank you, Jack, for all our long hours of amazing conversations, and simply being a great guy.

v

For my son, Zack Marroso, my guy.

A GUY'S GUIDE
TO SEX FOR TEENS
AND THEIR PARENTS!

Why is a guy's guide to sex so important? Secretly, guys need and want a guide to girls and sex. A teenage guy isn't going to ask for it, he isn't going to even pretend he wants it, but in his life, every day, he is wondering what to do when it comes to girls and sex. Not a day goes by that a teenage guy doesn't have questions, and need answers, about sex and relationships. Secretly. Most parents want to have "The Talk" with their teenage son, and they know they need to talk to him about sex, too. Yet, even the best of parents find it very challenging to talk to their teenager about everything they need to know, and knowing what to say or how to say it. The truth is most teenage guys aren't open to talking to their parents about sex or STDs or dating or even talking to girls. It would probably be easier to get your son to volunteer to mow the lawn or even paint the entire house, than talk frankly and openly about sex, right?

Most teenagers don't want to talk to their parents about sex, and most parents don't feel comfortable talking with their teens about sex, either. Chances are "The Talk" isn't going to last very long or give parents the chance to tell their son what they want him to know about relationships and sexuality, to be safe and healthy. As a sex therapist, I hear from parents that call and ask about their teenager after a crisis, such as finding their 15-year-old son in their bed naked with his 14-year-old, under-the-age-of-consent girlfriend, when they came home from work early one day. Or finding out that he was downloading pornography from the Internet. The parent gets scared and calls frantically asking, "What do I do?" The answer is to talk with him about sex or give him a guide to healthy sexuality, that includes information on more sexual topics than they would have covered or considered in a lifetime of talks, or both.

For some parents, the answer is to tell their teenager to stay away from having any sexual activity. Many parents tell their children to not have sex, to choose abstinence, just say no to sex, and save sex for marriage. Like many vows of abstinence, sexual abstinence vows are often eventually broken, and the majority of teenagers will engage in sexual behavior, whether they are prepared to be sexually safe or not. In every country around the globe, teenagers do have sexual relationships. By the time in America boys reach the age of 18, 63% of teens have been sexually active; by age 20, there is over 80% probability of teens engaging in sex. Worldwide, the majority of teens are sexually active by the time they are 20 years old. Whether one is a teen or waits until marriage to be sexually active, most adults do have sex for the first time sometime, and need guidance on how to be ready, responsible and safe.

The Truth About Guys and Sex

On Sex

- 82% of teen guys engage in sexual activity
- 10% of boys have had sexual intercourse by age 13

- 30% of boys have received oral sex by age 15
- 70% of boys have engaged in giving and/or receiving oral sex by age 19.
- Nearly 5% of teen boys have same sex sexual experiences

On Pregnancy

- 1 in 12 teens get pregnant *every* year
- 1 in 5 sexually active teens gets pregnant
- 33% of teen boys do not use condoms
- 90% of girls who don't use birth control get pregnant within a year
- 33% of teen pregnancies end in abortion

On Sexually Transmitted Diseases

- 1 out of 4 teens gets an STD
- 25% of new AIDS cases are young people under 21 years old
- 50% of new AIDS cases are young people under 25

(alanguttmacher.org, 2006, Division of Vital Statistics, 2005)

As a parent of a teenage son, a sex therapist and sex researcher, knowing what I know about teenage sexuality, I have two major concerns for teenagers. My number one concern is the high health risk for getting an STD, a sexually transmitted disease. As many as 25% of guys get an STD. If one third of guys are not using condoms, and a fourth of their sexual partners have an STD, the risk of getting an STD is seriously scary. The truth is that teens often don't know they have an STD, and often don't have any physical symptoms of infection. So, they give it to someone unknowingly with sexual contact. Both girls and guys are at a high risk for contracting STDs in their teens and early 20's, but many still do not use any protection against contracting diseases, including AIDs. Young men, especially those experimenting in same sex behaviors, which even some heterosexual guys do when they are teenagers, are at a high risk for AIDS. Even when teenagers claim sexual abstinence, over 50% are in engaging in oral sex, both giving and receiving it, which is not safe sex—you can get STDs from any exchange of bodily fluids. A recent study in Great Britain discovered that 74% of guys did not know you could get an STD from oral sex performed on a girl (http://alanguttmacher.org/media/nr/2006/03/15/index.html).

My number two concern is teenage pregnancy. With one third of guys not using condoms, and 90% of teen girls getting pregnant without any birth control use, the concern of pregnancy is real. The good news is that pregnancy rates have decreased in the last 10 years, mostly due to delaying sex and an increased use of birth control.

> Sex education does, indeed, teach teens to delay sex or act responsibly to avoid unwanted pregnancy!

Still, American teenagers have the highest pregnancy, childbirth and abortion rate than any other developed country! Why? For one, American teens are less likely to have sex education that teaches how to use reliable methods of birth control, and many teens have no way to get birth control, either. A lot of parents and schools primarily stress sexual abstinence, and they don't want to talk about any alternatives, for when teenagers do become sexually active. In some cases, parents think that schools provide sex education. Yet, many schools can not even talk about contraception in schools! Many schools are severely restricted in teaching about anything but abstinence, oh, unless you have already had a baby! Now that is like closing the barn door after the horse is out, isn't it?

So, why do guys need a guide for sex? Guys need guidance to make the right choices, right from the start, and keep making choices about sex from the first time to the next time and every time. Sex is not a single choice about the first time or about losing your virginity, it involves choices people make in a part of their life that will be with them all of their life. Even if one makes sexual mistakes, which a lot of guys in this book have made, they can always learn to make safer, healthier choices about life by making better decisions in the future.

Virgin Sex is about giving guys information to avoid getting hurt by sex, both emotionally and physically: to avoid making sexual mistakes that can cost them their lives or change their lives forever.

Sexual experiences, situations, and consequences shape the lives and the future of teenagers—our sons and daughters, our friends, our brothers, nephews, and grandsons! As a sex therapist, I know what is really going on with teens and sex today, and I'm sure most parents would want their sons to know what they need to know to be safe, sexually speaking. Guys need a guide *before* they try out their sexual ideas. Just like teens need driver's training *before* they get behind the wheel of a car, teens need sexual information *before* they start having closer, sexual relationships. Driver's education gives you a good foundation of knowledge about driving, signs, cars, directions, how to work the controls, and defensively driving so that reckless drivers don't hurt them. Teens use a few short weeks of education in driver's ed as a foundation of knowledge for their whole life. Guys need at least a few short weeks of education as a guide for sex, too.

When is the right time? Every state has different laws on what age is the right age to be able to legally drive. The average age is 15 or 16. Some teens are ready to take the wheel of a car at 15. But, many aren't. Even though they are legally able to drive, some parents won't let them get a beginner's permit or let them get a license, until they can show they are more responsible, like getting good grades, or following the rules in the home. Parents can be there and make that choice for kids about when they think their child is old enough to take on the responsibility to drive. Parents can have their kids pass tests, both written and driving tests, to prove that they are ready to drive and take their life into their own hands, and be responsible for others' lives.

How does a parent know when it is the time to put a kid into driving lessons? Some parents take their kids out driving at 12 or 13, long before it is "legal" to try to drive, usually on a farm or some back country roads or even the high school parking lot which is empty late at night or in the summer. How does a parent know when? Usually because a kid is asking to try it! "Let me hold the wheel"; "Let me back the car out of the driveway"; "When are you going to teach me to drive?" Teens, especially guys, won't ask parents "When are you going to tell me about sex?"; "Let me tell you about kissing a girl at school"; "When can I start having sex?" Yet, long before it is "legal" for teens to have sex, at the age of consent, which might be age 16 (on average) or later, teens do take the "car out for a drive," and experiment sexually. Twenty-five percent of middle school kids have sexual experiences, through sexual touching and oral sex.

Parents can't always be there for teens when it comes to relationships and sex. Yet, sex education and guidance can never be taken away and can always be heard in one's mind, if it is taught. Parents don't give kids lessons on driving *after* they've wrecked the car: they give them lessons before an accident happens. Although knowledge won't prevent all accidents, it can prevent some, to learn to steer clear of dangerous situations and how to act in them when they happen, to prevent them again in the future. When the time or situations arises where the sex drive is in gear, teens can be equipped to handle the road of relationships, some which will have sexual pitstops.

By using the Dr. Darcy's "Are you Ready for Sex?" Quiz in Chapter Four, any parent can talk to their teens about sex, encouraging them to avoid sex until they can "pass" all the conditions needed to be ready for a sexual relationship. Parents might not be able to make their teens pass a test to be ready for sex, but they can give them the quiz as a guide to make the right decisions in a sexual situation or relationship. This guide isn't just a one time test one takes for a license to have sex the rest of their lives, it is a guide to use now and for the rest of their lives, when they are thinking about whether or not they are ready for sex in a particular situation, with a particular person, and at a particular time in their life. Discussing the questions in the quiz also gives you a chance to share your values about sexuality.

When is the right time to give your teens a guide to sex? Before they have sexual touch, before they share oral sex, before they get someone pregnant, and before they get emotionally hurt by making sexual mistakes or before the next time or the next sexual decision. Nine percent of guys are sexually assaulted or raped, and 25% of girls are raped by guys. Guys need to know the rules on sexual touch and learn to get permission for sex, to avoid any misunderstandings about sex. Chapter Nine outlines specific ways to avoid sexual assault, before it happens, which is very important for every guy. In societies where sexuality is openly spoken of, freely discussed, joyously explained and experienced, there are very few sexual crimes, and only very small number of births occur unexpectedly. Yet, in our society, where sexual silence is considered appropriate when it comes to educating teenagers, many adults have sexual problems, and sex therapists are in almost every large city. Sexual secrets shape lives forever. Guys need to be able to talk openly about their sexual concerns, whether it is about sexual assault, first sexual feelings, how to know when it's OK to kiss a girl or go further, or knowing about a

A Guy's Guide to Sex for Teens and Their Parents!

girl's period. Guys need a guide to sex and relationships before they have sex to develop a happy, healthy foundation for sexuality for life: for themselves and their partners.

Guys also need a guide to understand girls and have relationships with girls, *before* they start having sexual relationships and as a part of having a sexual relationship. Some guys don't understand this until after they've already had sexual experiences, which can cause a lot of confusion and embarrassment, too. Some guys don't feel they have a problem with sex, except that they want to know how to have it with a girl, or more of it. A few years ago, I was doing a lecture on sexuality at the University of South Carolina. At the end of my speech, I invited anyone to ask "one free sex question" answered by a live sex therapist. A huge big-mouthed football player, as cocky as the Carolina Gamecocks mascot, burst out yelling, "Yeah, how do I get more sex?" I paused, letting the loud laughter quiet down, smiled and said, "The answer is simple: You have more quality and you'll get more quantity." Suddenly, the puffed up roaring linebacker shrunk back into his seat, mumbling, "Uh, yeah, ok." Obviously, this guy needed to learn a lot more about getting along with girls, which is discussed throughout this book, including sexual communication, which is needed to have a sexual relationship of any quality.

This book is written for guys, some who are still virgins and some who are teens and inexperienced but sexually active young men. *Virgin Sex* is a real sex education, using true stories from boys to men to give them a guide to healthy sexuality for life. Knowledge is power. It is the key to unlocking the mystery of understanding girls and women. As a sex therapist, and as a woman, I am going to give guys a foundation of sexual knowledge, straight from the couch of a sex therapist, to provide them with information needed to be the best they can be when it comes to relationships and sex. For example, one of the greatest and worst myths is that sex for the first time for girls has to hurt: girls and guys both buy into this very damaging myth. This book helps to destroy that myth, so that girls don't have to get hurt physically when they lose their virginity, and guys will know what to do to avoid inflicting pain on someone they love. First, guys can learn to treat a girl right, then learn the basics of sexual relationships, to begin having life-long relationships with girls and women. Quality does mean more quantity. Quantity will not be a question: every girl wants a good guy.

> When it comes to sex: The good guys finish first, and they get seconds, too!

This book will share real, true stories of guys' relationships and sexual experiences, with advice on how to get lucky with girls. Guys will learn that luck has a lot to do with skill and practice, just like in sports or other pursuits. My goal in writing this book is to help you guys understand girls, how to avoid getting hurt by the mean girls, as well as learn about sex. A lot of girls get hurt by guys, both emotionally and physically, and get hurt by sex, too. Most guys do not want to hurt girls, but they often do. These negative experiences can scar girls, and some guys, too, and turn them off to sex for life. Remember, these girls are going to grow up to be your classmates, girlfriends, wives, and mothers of your children. When most girls are treated right, they will do anything to please you and try to make you happy. Girls that get hurt by guys and relationships and sex don't trust guys and can learn to hate sex. Yes, it's amazing, but every week women come into my office because they don't like sex, even when they love their boyfriends or husbands. Sometimes men don't like sex because of bad experiences they've had with women. A grown man's worst nightmare is to feel trapped, being married to someone who hates sex and doesn't trust men. If every guy learned how to treat girls right, emotionally and sexually, it is more likely that when these girls grow up and become your girlfriends or wives, they will have a happy foundation for sexuality, so you can share in healthy sexuality together. *Virgin Sex for Guys* will teach you how to be a great guy, a great friend, a great lover, and one day enjoy one of the greatest gifts on Earth: to love and be loved.

xviii

ONE

WHY GUYS THINK THEY WANT SEX—OR NOT

1

This is the real talk about sex, just for guys. Beyond "the talk" from your parents, way more than you've learned from your buddies, and past the fallopian tubes talk in school, this is the truth from a real sex therapist. Most young men don't know how to talk to girls and they don't understand women. Actually, a lot of older men don't either, so don't feel bad or alone. Cluelessness from guys is one of the reasons many guys and girls get hurt by sex. It's not that it's easy: girls are hard to understand. And to make it tougher, girls change all the time. Once you finally figure out how to get along with a girl and seemingly, be happy, she changes her mind and wants something else. A strong message in *Virgin Sex for Girls* is for girls to develop a "sexual voice." A sexual voice means speaking up about what you want and don't want when it comes to your sexuality. Generally, girls are taught not to say what they want for a lot of different reasons, one being to please their boyfriends or to go along with whatever is happening, so they'll be liked. Without a sexual voice, a lot of girls get hurt by sex, and sometimes a guy doesn't even know it!

Guys don't usually have as much of a problem saying what they want, sexually speaking, but you guys need to develop a sexual voice, too. Learning to communicate is a very important part of being in a relationship, especially in a sexual relationship, not only for yourself and for your needs, but to understand your partner and what they like. Short of getting your information from the clue fairy, you can learn to talk to girls, find out what they want, and unravel the mystery of happy, fun relationships. One of the first decisions you have to make about sex is answering the question, "Why do I want to have sex?" If you think the answer is simple, like, "Duh, because I am a guy!" then you will learn a lot from reading about what other guys who also thought that when they experienced sex to just have sex. First, thinking about why you want to experience sex, with whom, in what circumstance, and putting thought behind your behavior is the first step to not making your first sexual mistake. In Chapter Two, you will learn the "Top Ten Sexual Mistakes That Guys Make." The first mistake is to have sex with the first girl who says yes. This chapter will help you to begin thinking about your reasons for having sex—or not.

To Lose My Virginity—Rusty's Story

Rusty's goal, when he turned 15 was "to get laid." On his 15th birthday, after the presents were opened and the cake was eaten and the ice cream was still melting on the island in the kitchen, his Dad asked him, "So, what are your dreams and goals in life, for your 15th year?" Rusty was shameless: he told his dad, right in front of his older sister and younger brother, "Lose my virginity."

Now, Rusty hadn't ever done anything more than kiss a girl. One kiss, to be exact. He fell in love once, just 2 months earlier, when he was 14, with a girl he talked to mostly on the phone. After several phone calls, she freaked out when he professed his eternal love to her and asked her to profess her love to him. As you can see, Rusty was clueless when it came to love and sex. All he knew was that he was madly, intensely in love with this girl that he'd only seen in person twice. Abruptly, in the middle of one of his pleading phone calls, asking Bethany for her promise of love to him, her mom got on the phone and told him directly that he was freaking out her daughter and to quit calling and leave Bethany alone. Rusty was very embarrassed and never called again.

This was the extent of Rusty's experience with girls. Rusty was a virgin, but he was shameless in his desire to lose his virginity, and he continued his desperate pursuit throughout the year [which we'll read about later]. Despite his first love rejection, he still knew that he wanted one thing: to have sex!

Desperation is a very unpleasant aftershave. Rusty was bathed in it, and it stank! Girls can smell desperation from a mile away, and even as much as they would love to have a boyfriend, a clingy, possessive guy who just wants to have sex is a big turn off!

Needless to say, you guessed it, Rusty did not "get laid" in his 15th year. He did manage to make out with a girl once, with whom he fell madly in love, like Bethany. He called her and called her and begged her to have sex. Again, his desperation totally turned that girl off, too, and he made a big fool of himself.

Rusty had a lot to learn about girls, like most guys who have no idea of where to start, and no idea of how to get to the "finish line." *Virgin Sex for Guys* is to help guys like Rusty, and guys like you know where to begin with girls, how to avoid making a fool out of yourself, and give you the confidence to relate to girls, too.

In Love—John's Story

John met Cissy when he was 15, almost 16. They started out as friends, hanging out and talking. For about 3 months, he really liked her and he wanted to go out with her. He started telling her that they should go out and that he really liked her. She was hesitant to go out with him, but he was persistent. He kept going to places she was going and hanging out with her, then talking to her. He kind of con-

3

vinced her, with her finally agreeing, to "try to be his girlfriend."

John went out with Cissy for 4 years. He was totally in love with her. She fell totally in love with him. They were great friends. He learned how to be a boyfriend: to call her every day or talk to her every day and he loved it! He was totally into her and he wanted to see her all the time.

At first, they kissed and hugged and hung out watching movies on the couch, hanging all over each other. Then they started making out, which turned into big time messing around. Gradually, they felt comfortable being naked together and lying around in his bed and messing around, but they didn't have sex until 3 years after their relationship started. Cissy was kind of quiet and shy and she just didn't want to have sex yet. She wanted to save sex for the guy she was going to marry.

One time, when they were big time messing around, it just happened! John was lying on top of her and they were pressed together and his penis just slipped into Cissy's vagina. They both were surprised, a little freaked out, and stopped. They got up and talked about it. They just sat down and talked about having sexual intercourse together, as a part of their relationship. Both of them were very much in love, and they were both virgins. The whole situation with them messing around and "it just happening" accidentally was O.K. after they talked. John says he was very considerate and reassuring to Cissy, and didn't pressure her to go ahead with a sexual relationship. Cissy and John both agreed they wanted to share their virginity with each other, and they planned it. John got condoms and they planned a special day and made love for the first time. They were both 19. They even got engaged a little while later.

A year or so later, John lost a lot of weight. He had been a pretty heavy kid and was 60 pounds overweight. He went on a serious diet and lost all the extra weight. He started getting a lot of looks and attention from girls. Cissy started getting jealous and starting accusing him of cheating. John swears he never cheated, not once, not even a kiss, not ever. He loved Cissy, but he couldn't convince her that

**she could trust him. The trust issue became a constant fight and they
ended breaking up. Actually, they ended up getting back together
a few times, but by that time, they had different friends and it just
didn't work. Nevertheless, John has absolutely no regrets about his
first sexual experiences. In fact, he has a lot of really wonderful,
sweet memories.**

John really was in love with Cissy. He waited three years to have
sexual intercourse with her, although they made out a lot before
they actually lost their virginity. Cissy just wasn't ready for "going all
the way," and John understood and accepted her feelings. It wasn't
like John was this perfect kid: he was pretty much a hellraiser, in
fact. He smoked weed and drank beer and messed up in school and
drove his mom crazy at times. He drove his friends' parents crazy,
too. But, when it came to his girlfriend, he really loved her and cared
about her and waited until she was ready for sex.

Guys have a reputation for wanting and having sex if they can
get it, whenever the first or any opportunity, deemed a lucky opportunity, presents itself. So, if a young man is not sexually active
or lucky enough to have a girlfriend to mess around with, it must be
because he has not been lucky enough to, well, "get laid."

As a result, every girl thinks every guy wants to have sex. In fact,
it *is* true that every girl hears that every guy just wants to have sex,
sounding something like "that's all guys are after is sex."

So, if you are one of these guys who is still a virgin, at say 15,
18, or 23, there must be a mortal flaw with you, right? It must mean
that you're unpopular, unattractive, awkward, and unable to get girlfriends. Right? Wrong!

Some guys who are still virgins, when it seems like all their
friends are talking about their sexual conquests, would like to lose
their virginity as soon as possible. Some guys choose to wait until it
is right for them, for a lot of reasons. One of the reasons might be a
vow to be abstinent until they are married. Later on, we'll talk about

Why Guys Think They Want Sex—or Not

abstinence and religious reasons for waiting to have sex. For now, the most important factor in deciding about being sexually active, is that it is the right decision for you. Chapter Four talks about how to know if you're ready for sex, depending on your values, your family, your relationship, and what you want.

What *is* true is that a lot of guys think about girls and would love to know how to talk to girls and how to get a girlfriend. A lot of guys also think it would be great to try having sex and see what it is like, but they don't even know what it is like to have a relationship, let alone mess around in a sexual way. Chapter Two will give you a lot of great info on how to talk to girls and treat girls right, which will help you understand and get along with girls better.

John's advice for guys is: Wait until you find someone you really care about and that makes all the difference!

The Knight-In-Shining Armor Syndrome—Charlie C's Story

Charlie C. had his first sexual experience with a girl at 15. When he was 13 and 14, he had a lot of girlfriends with whom he would kiss and hug and make-out. Sometimes he was going with a girl for a little while, sometimes he was just talking to a girl and they would end up kissing and making out. He got into a lot of middle school arguments when he got in between two girls. He would be kissing and hanging out with one girl, and the next week talking and doing the same with another and then they would talk and they'd get mad and he was in the middle, feeling stupid. Girls jealously talking to each other taught him a lot. He decided to stick with one girl after that, and treat them right.

At 15, Charlie was working in a restaurant. He was a busboy

and "Jackie" was a busgirl. They worked together, they hung out after work, and they were friends. He was a virgin, she wasn't. She asked him to have sex. They had messed around, kissing and making out, sometimes really hot and heavy, but they never had sex. Jackie asked Charlie to have sex with her. Charlie didn't feel it was right. He wanted to be sensitive and understanding and he didn't want to pressure her or push her for sex. He didn't want her to feel like she "had to" do it. Really, he wanted to make sure it was really O.K. and he didn't want her to regret it. He thought a lot about her feelings and the "big picture," and how having sex with him might "change her."

Charlie loved Jackie. He liked her and he loved her. Even though it was deep for his age, he thought about how sex "on a soul" level affected girls and made them become more attached and he just wanted to really make sure it was O.K. with her.

Jackie had been hurt in her life. He father had died in a car accident a few years earlier. He was drunk and he hit a tree and died. Jackie had never been the same since then: she was a daddy's girl and she missed her father terribly. Jackie had suffered from depression from time to time ever since the accident.

Jackie reminded Charlie that he wasn't her first. In fact, she told him she had been through the whole guy pressuring her thing, knew what that was like, but she certainly didn't feel that way with him. They ended up having sex for the first time for Charlie and it was great, really great. Even when Jackie went around telling other girls that she'd had sex with Charlie, and told them he was "hung like a horse," it didn't bother him too much, or "it didn't hurt my ego anyway."

What did hurt was the break-up.

Jackie said the "L" word. She told Charlie she loved him. Charlie felt like he loved her back and he told her! Then, Charlie didn't hear from her for 3 weeks. He didn't even see her at work: she just stopped showing up. Charlie felt very hurt and wondered what had happened to Jackie. He just didn't understand. After a couple of weeks of unanswered phone calls, Charlie finally went to her mother to ask what happened to her. Her mother said she was depressed and she started doing drugs and hanging out with wild kids: bikers, stoners, rough kids. Her mom felt real bad, but told Charlie it just wasn't his fault, he was a good guy, and what Jackie was doing was wrong.

Charlie moved on, although his heart was torn up for a little while. It especially hurt when he found out she had had a three-some with his brother and another girl, but he never understood why. She had also become promiscuous (slept with a lot of guys) after they broke up.

Charlie C. was a good guy. He tried to be a great guy when it came to Jackie and sex. He really thought about her feelings and wanting sex to be O.K. for her. He realized that a lot of girls regretted sex and he didn't want to be one of those guys who pushed himself on girls, and then they regretted it later.

Nevertheless, Jackie was a wild girl. She had a lot of family problems. She had a major problem really attaching herself to a guy and being in love. She also had a problem with drugs and depression.

Charlie didn't regret his first sexual experience, but he did get hurt by her just running away and never talking to him about it. He just didn't understand why his love for her couldn't save her. He thought about them having a future together and being together a long time. He was dreaming and it was a fantasy he made up all on his own. In truth, he realized that he was trying to rescue Jackie from her past and her pain, but he couldn't do it. She was a hurt girl, who needed a lot of help, more than his love could heal.

After that, he tried to be around girls who didn't have so many problems, problems that were way over his head to handle. He stopped trying to rescue girls, at least as much.

A few years later, Charlie ran into Jackie at a gas station she was working at, nearby his work. She never said why she ran away from love. Charlie figured she got scared about falling in love and she was afraid to attach herself to someone and lose them again, like she lost her dad. Charlie had begged her not to do drugs when they were together. He knew she had been into drugs, since her daddy died, and he told her she didn't need to do drugs when she was with him. She had a "death wish." She hung out with a rough crowd and wore a black bandana, with white skulls and crossbones all over it. Some more years past, and Charlie found out she died. She was high on drugs and ran her car into a tree, dying the same way her daddy died.

Sadly, many guys think they can be the knight in shining armor on a white horse and save the girl. In truth, the girl has to save herself first, before she will let you love her in any way. Girls will push you away and make it very hard to just "love them the right way." Love doesn't have to be that hard. Read that sentence again: Love doesn't have to be that hard. There is nothing wrong with being sensitive and understanding to girls and thinking of their feelings, first. In fact, it can make you a great man! BUT: Get off your horse, come down to earth and find someone who can love and give like you want to love and give.

Charlie's advice to guys: Love first. Be loved. If you aren't, being a savior can make you a victim.

To Prove I Wasn't a Virgin — Tyrell's Story

Tyrell was 14. He had a two older cousins, around 16 and 17. They hung out all the time in the neighborhood, where their families lived. Tyrell bragged to his cousins that he was not a virgin. Of course, he didn't give out any names or details, but he assured his cousin that "no way—I am not a virgin." His cousins were not convinced, but they didn't tell him that at the time.

His cousins set up a situation with an older girl, who was known to be very easy. The cousins knew her real well, and all three of them went over to the girl's house, when her mama wasn't home, to hang out. The cousins brought up the fact that they thought Tyrell was a virgin, which he still denied. Apparently, the girl had a thing about wanting to "take a guy's virginity," and she agreed to have sex with Tyrell—right then and there.

The girl just told Tyrell to come over to the couch and she would "help him." Tyrell, of course, felt like he had to, although he was extremely uncomfortable in the situation. Secretly, Tyrell was thinking he wanted to wait until he was married to have sex, like his preacher and mom taught him in church. He just ran his mouth to fit in with his older cousins. Now, Tyrell was caught: he could admit he was a liar, or he could go along with it and prove his manhood. He felt like he just couldn't be a liar about his manhood, so he had to prove it.

Tyrell not only had never had sex, but he had never masturbated or ejaculated before. He was taught it was a sin to "touch himself down there," so he hadn't (except to go to the bathroom, of course).

Tyrell went over to the couch. He pulled down his pants. His cousins were on the other side of the room—watching T.V. but they were kind of watching, too. It was really uncomfortable, but Tyrell felt he had to prove himself and live up to his lies or be caught in them. He got hard and he put his penis inside her, with her help. He didn't even wear a condom, which was really worrying him. As soon as she touched him, he began to feel a very strange sensation! He felt his whole body shaking. His back jerked, his pelvis lurched, and he got flushed hot all over, like an instant fever. Then, he got scared, and he screamed out loud—very loud, thinking he was going to die and also going straight to hell. At the same time, he felt like

**there was an explosion coming out his penis. He was afraid that he
urinated right on this girl and he screamed again in fear and embarrassment. Then he pulled up his pants and he ran out the house. All
he could hear was the girl and his cousins laughing and howling. He
was never more embarrassed in his life—then or ever since.**

Tyrell was a 14-year-old guy, who was running his mouth, afraid
to let people know he was a virgin, and he had sex just to disprove
his lies. Tyrell stayed away from sex after that for a long time. He
really regretted going against his religious values and he even went
to confession at church the next Sunday. It took years to live down
his embarrassment, because his cousins teased him about it for a very
long time. Tyrell didn't have sex with another girl until after he finished high school and left home, and after he fell in love with the
girl first. He wishes he had not lied and bragged and set himself up
for being a fool, but now he laughs about it.

11

Tyrell's advice for guys: Wait until you find someone
that it means something to be with. It is definitely
worth the wait. Also, don't be ashamed about being
a virgin, and: Don't LIE! Don't be afraid to stand up
and say, I'm waiting until it means something important to me.

Guys who are really your friends will respect you for saying that.
Guys who really care about you will understand. Guys who don't
even know you that well will admire you for your individuality and
strength. It might be really hard to stand up for what you want, but,
trust me and trust yourself: it will be better in the long run.

She Said Yes—Ryan's Story

Ryan was 14, and in 9th grade. He had been thinking about having sex for about two years. He felt like he was just like most of his guy friends in middle school, who thought they were pretty cool guys, when in fact, they hung out with each other at the lunch table and school and they just looked at the girls hanging out at their lunch table at school. They sat on the opposite sides of the cafeteria, pretending not to look over at each other and laugh and gossip about each other. Yes, says Ryan, guys are big gossipers, too.

Ryan said the guys gossip about sports and school and what friends got in trouble and stuff, but also which girls were putting out. Secretly, Ryan would watch the girls go by and think: which girls were virgins and which ones weren't? Ryan didn't even like any one girl, he was looking for just one to like him. Ryan was waiting for that note in class where someone would tell him that someone kind of, maybe, sort of, or definitely liked him. In fact, he dreamed about it and he fantasized about it. As of the end of middle school, that note never came, and he didn't send one, either. He was too afraid, even when he thought a girl was really cute or hot, he never sent the note, nor did he get a friend to do it for him—he was too cool for that. He was not going to be one of those weird geeks who goes all ga-ga over a girl, then gets laughed at the next day at the lunch table in the cafeteria. Nope, he was just too good for that. Or maybe he had too much pride.

The summer before high school started out pretty uneventful. His parents both worked and he was home alone, with a list of chores and a pool to take care of, too. For the first couple of weeks of summer, most of his friends were on family trips or at camp and he didn't do much. Then he started going over to a neighborhood pool where one of his friends was working and he could get in for free. That's where he started hanging out with Casey. Casey was considered a "ho" (short for whore). She was one of those girls who got talked about a lot in the cafeteria at school. She had huge breasts and everyone said she was easy. Ryan had heard that she gave 2 different guys oral sex and had sex with a guy who was going to college next year.

Actually, Ryan kind of didn't want to get caught talking to her, since she had a bad reputation. But during the week, there weren't that many people from school at the pool, just a lot of moms with little kids. So, when the pool was not too busy, he started going over and talking to Casey. At first, he'd pretend like he was swimming near her when she was in the water and bump into her "by mistake." After a couple of times of doing that, he finally walked by her lounge chair and said he was sorry and said hi.

Casey really wasn't like what he thought she would be like. She was nice. She was funny, really funny, and made him laugh. She would go to the pool by herself and do her "summer reading" on the deck. Ryan was going to be in her same English class level the next year, so he started out by asking her to tell him a blow-by-blow of the books chapters, thinking then he wouldn't have to read it himself. Actually, he started liking her. He started looking forward to going to the pool and talking to her. At the same time, he was a little embarrassed to be seen talking to her, which he feels guilty about now.

One day, he got up the nerve to ask her if she had a boyfriend. She said no. Well, that conversation didn't go too far. He really wanted to know if all the rumors about her were true. The next day, he asked her if she'd ever had a boyfriend. She told him about hanging out with the guy who was going to college, then she started crying. Ryan felt really uncomfortable and didn't really know what to do. He just sat there and finally asked her why she was crying. She told him that there were all these rumors that she and that college guy had had sex and they didn't, and her parents even heard about it and how horrible that was and all.

"GEEZ!" Ryan was thinking: "I just wanted to talk to her because maybe I could have sex with her because she's easy and here it all was a lie and now I even kind of like her! What the heck am I going to do?"

13

Then came the moment of truth. Casey asked Ryan if he had heard any of the rumors.

"OHMIGOD!" Ryan thought. Lying was his first thought. Definitely, I should lie! Then the thought of the 6th or 7th or 8th commandment came to his head and he was repeating in his mind, "Thou shalt not bear false witness." Then, he thought he should just lie and get it over with anyway.

Finally, he said: "Yeah, I did hear that at the cafeteria at school— but, but I didn't believe it!" OK, that was a half lie. Actually, he was hoping it was true that she had sex with the college guy, so he could have a chance, a half a chance to maybe have sex this summer. Now, here she was this really pretty nice girl, crying over rumors that he helped to spread, and it turns out, *she's a virgin,* and his chances with her were probably out the window forever.

Casey turned from a kind of nice girl to a psycho girl, screaming "Who was it? Who was spreading all those rumors! Was it Stevie B.?"

Ryan's eyes got huge. He became mute. He says he really lost his voice. He couldn't speak. He was tagged. Ryan's guilt got the best of him and when he got his voice back, one word at a time, it seemed, he told her the truth: exactly who said what, when, where, and how. He was roped in by his growing feelings for Casey, of love and pity combined.

After that whole scene at the pool, Ryan went home figuring his now active fantasy life with Casey for a summer of fun was over. He avoided the pool for a day, then a couple of days, then a week. He hung out with some guy friends for a few days, and had some fun, but he found himself actually missing talking to Casey. A week later, he went back to the pool. Sure enough, Casey was there, reading the second of their summer reading books, which he hadn't even started yet, as usual. This time, she came up to him. She said she was sorry for going off on him and she was just upset over all the rumors, but she was pretty much over it.

After that, Ryan started really hanging out with Casey. After a couple of weeks, they started secretly hanging out at his house, when his parent's were at work. They became friends. They started making out and really, just having fun watching T.V. and playing video games at his house. She even helped him clean the pool, so he wouldn't get in trouble when his parents came home. She never did offer him oral sex, which was his total fantasy, given her "reputation." He finally figured out that that was all a bunch of lies, too. Casey said that "girls with big tits are always thought to be sluts, but I'm not." After that, they became boyfriend and girlfriend and spent the rest of the summer together. Later that summer, Ryan and Casey talked about having sex for the first time. He asked, she said yes.

Ryan's story has a twist. You think he was just going to be having easy sex with that easy girl who said yes to him. However, Ryan found out the hard way that rumors aren't usually true, and they hurt girls, too. Casey said yes, eventually, because they became good friends and learned to like each other, for who they really were. Casey was funny, fun, and hot, too. Ryan was awkward, kind of geeky, but really had his luck with Casey when he got real and told her the truth about stuff as her friend.

Ryan's advice for guys: Don't believe all the rumors you hear about girls. Don't assume just because a girl has a great body that every guy is doing her. Remember, there's a person in there, and she might be nice.

My Golden Opportunity with the Hottest Girl in School — Jon's Story

Jon came in for sex therapy when he was 18. He had tried to have sex three times with this beautiful girl, Amber, but he couldn't. Jon thought Amber was just the hottest girl at school, but he really didn't have any feelings for her emotionally. When he finally got his chance to be with her, he couldn't get an erection! In his words, Jon whispered to me, embarrassed, "No matter what I did, my dick just wouldn't get hard!" First, Jon thought about going to get Viagra (a prescription drug generally for older men who have problems with erections), but he decided to talk to a sex therapist instead.

Jon was talking to a lot of girls and was dating a girl other than Amber, although they weren't in an exclusive relationship. When he was having sex with his girlfriend, Jon didn't have any problems, but Jon was very worried because he really found Amber to be so beautiful: she had one of the hottest bodies he had ever seen. He really was excited to be with her and more excited when she asked him to have sex with her. Amber was 17 and was a virgin. She wanted to give her virginity to Jon. She didn't even care for Jon that much; she just felt that she was not only ready for sex but wanted to lose her virginity, to try sex, with him. Jon couldn't have been more excited, but when it came to actually having sexual intercourse, Jon just couldn't "get it up." He just didn't understand what was wrong with him and he was worried about his performance and his reputation.

Sex is more than just the functions of the body. Every person has his or her own "conditions for sex." For some people, that means being married. For some people, that means being in love. For others, it is having an available sexual partner to whom they are attracted in some way. For Jon, finding out that he really didn't like Amber that much was sufficient to put a damper on his physical desire for her. That is, he found her physically beautiful, but he didn't have any loving feelings for her. When it came down to it, he felt guilty about "making love" and "taking her virginity" when he knew he wasn't in love with her or wasn't "the one" for whom she was looking.

Jon found out the hard (or soft) way that one of his "conditions" for enjoying sex was that he had to have emotional feelings for someone and he couldn't just be satisfying someone else, or satisfying his own physical urges for that matter. In Chapter Four, in "How to Know if You're Ready for Sex," we'll talk about your "conditions" for sex. Conditions are what you need and value and want before you have a sexual relationship. Jon didn't know about his conditions and he felt really badly about himself at first, because he saw himself as this big sexual stud-muffin who could do anything, any time, any way to please someone, but he couldn't. Jon was a human being with human emotions. He needed to learn to respect that about himself, to respect the wisdom of his penis, as it were, and learn his conditions for lovemaking. Also, he realized he should respect his body and not even *think* of taking Viagra to overrule his body's emotions.

Girls Pressured ME—Sammy's Story

Sammy lived with his mom after his parents divorced when he was little, until he was 14. He spent every other weekend with his Dad, and Christmas and summer vacations, and he had a stepsister in his same grade. Sammy got along with kids at school, but he never had any real friends outside of school, because his mom didn't like much company at their house. He didn't know the first thing about really talking to girls.

On the weekends, Sammy liked staying with his stepsister. She had a lot of friends in his Dad's neighborhood and over time, they became Sammy's friends, too. Finally, at 14, Sammy convinced his mom to let him go live with his dad, stepmom, and his stepsister full time. After a few months, Sammy turned 15 and could drive, and his dad got him an awesome car: an older fire red sportscar that had a new engine, to drive to school. His new life was off to a great start!

Sammy was popular at his new school. He was good looking, nice, and was good at talking with girls. Mostly, he listened to his stepsister, who gave him all kinds of advice, but mostly taught him to just "be friends" with girls and get comfortable with just hanging out. Also, his stepmom was easy to talk to and she didn't mind having friends over at their house.

Sammy found out that being friends with girls was pretty easy, just talking and listening about all their guy problems and family problems, without any pressure about sex. Sammy found that girls liked that a lot and it helped him became popular.

In 10th grade, Sammy got a huge crush on a girl a year older than him, Sarah, when he was 15. She was 16. Sammy was only going out with her for 3 weeks and she asked him if he wanted a "blow job." He was a little bit surprised and said no. He told her, "Hey, you don't have to do that, just because we're going out." Well, after talking and another offer, he thought: "Sure, why not?" Of course, it was great! After a couple more weeks, his girlfriend asked him to have sex with him. Sammy started freaking. He didn't think he was ready to have sex. But, he wasn't sure, "I mean, why not?" But, Sammy was kind of scared about what if she got pregnant and all. So, he turned her offer of sex down. Actually, he told her he thought they should be going out longer than 3 weeks before they had sex and he wanted to get to know each other better. He really liked her and everything, but the sexual pressure was too sudden. At the same time, his girlfriend complained that he was too "touchy-feely." So, he told her that if he was too touchy-feely and she didn't like it, why would she want to have sex? Nevertheless, she still wanted to have sex with him and she was mad at him for not having sex with her. Finally, Sammy broke up with her, because she was rushing into things too fast.

After that, Sammy was not at all into just going out with one girl. He didn't want to have his heart broken again after having such a huge crush and feeling so hurt and rejected just because he wouldn't have sex with Sarah. Sammy found out that he didn't need to be in an exclusive relationship to have fun, make out, and even hook up to a certain extent with girls. In fact, over the next year, Sammy had at least 7 times when a girl offered to give him oral sex if he would be their boyfriend or even for no reason at all!

Sammy felt somewhat intimidated by so many aggressive girls coming after him and putting sexual demands on him. So, for a couple of years, he stayed away from any exclusive relationships. Sammy admits that a couple of times, he just couldn't turn oral sex down, especially when he really liked the girl and she was hot, too. But, really, Sammy didn't want to have a girlfriend because he didn't want to deal with a girlfriend. Sammy didn't like the obligation of having to call someone everyday, keep up with someone all the time and having a commitment. At least he told girls up front how he felt, and that he didn't want a "relationship." The summer before his senior year, Sammy became friends with one of his stepsister's friends, Lexie. Lexie was super sweet, cool, smart and was into things that he liked, and they hung out at his house a lot. Sammy had his first "real" sexual experience with Lexie.

Immediately, everyone knew what happened, because Lexie told his stepsister. Sammy's stepsister's other best friend, who had a really big mouth, told everyone because she had a crush on Sammy and she was jealous. After everyone found out, Sammy felt pretty uncomfortable and decided to just break up with Lexie, even though they were close. Sammy wasn't in love in Lexie and he didn't have a commitment to her, plus he just didn't want to deal with the drama.

At first, Sammy felt bad that he had sex with Lexie and then broke up with her soon afterwards. Sammy just felt like he couldn't deal with all the rumors and girl fighting that started over sex, especially since they were all fighting with his stepsister, in his own

19

Why Guys Think They Want Sex—or Not

house! Sex changed all their friendships, which Sammy wasn't expecting. Later, Sammy found out that Lexie had made a bet when Sammy first moved to town, on who would be the first one to have sex with him. Lexie won the $20 bet, and Sammy had been kind of used. In the long run, Sammy never felt too bad about being used, in fact, it was the other way around, but it made him feel less guilty for breaking up with her.

Sammy feels like his only love was with Sarah, and he has never felt the same way about another girl. He still has a special place in his heart for her. Because Sarah hurt him, he has problems with being committed and fears falling in love and getting hurt by girls. Also, Sammy saw a lot of conflict between his parents during and after the divorce that probably started his not really trusting relationships.

Sammy experienced a lot of situations with girls who were sexually aggressive. Some guys might read this and think, "Wow! I wish I had girls coming up to me and asking to give me a blow job!" Although it may sound like a fantasy, it was true, but for Sammy, as a 14-year-old, he wasn't at all prepared for relationships with girls. He hadn't had a lot of friendships because his mom never liked having anyone over at the house. When he moved to his Dad's house, he was overwhelmed with all the girls who wanted to go out with "the new guy in town." Sammy had fallen pretty fast for Sarah, but he was not ready for the sexual pressure she put on their relationship when they only knew each other for a very short time. Sammy is really glad he didn't just have sex with Sarah, but he did get hurt by her rejecting him and ridiculing him when he didn't go along with it. After Sarah, he had a lot more experiences with girls who were also sexually aggressive, even offering oral sex, just to have him be their boyfriend. Later, he did have sex for the first time with a girl he really did like and although he felt like she really liked him, too, he found out he was a part of a "bet" that she would have sex with him. Guys get bad reputations for playing "betting" or dare games about who will get who in the sack, but don't be fooled: girls can do this, too!

The truth is this: girls can be aggressive about sex. Most guys feel like they should be very overjoyed with this incredible opportunity to have "free sex," but a lot of guys feel intimidated and turned off by aggressive girls, too. A lot of guys feel insecure about themselves and uncertain about what they want to really do when it comes to having sexual relationships. Don't worry: this is very normal! Take it slowly. Wait. It is really OK and really very important to wait to have a sexual relationship until you are certain that it is "right." You may not be absolutely certain when it is right, but you will almost always be certain when it is wrong!

Why are some girls so aggressive about sex? A lot of times, and I think this was true for Sammy, girls think that if they have sex with a guy, the guy will like them. Some girls think sex is the only way they are ever going to have a boyfriend. Some girls feel they have to have sex, that sex is expected, and if they don't meet the expectations, they'll lose their boyfriend. Some girls, just as with guys, really don't know how to relate to guys and communicate with them, and they think it is easier to break the ice with sex to instantly get a guy to like them. For a small minority of girls, they just don't think sex is a big deal, and it is nothing to them to have sex. Believe it or not, with these girls, chances are pretty good that sex won't really be a big deal for you, either!

Sammy's advice to guys: Sharing your sexuality is more special when you share it with someone who is special to you.

FREE SEX: TRUTH OR DARE?

Don't let the idea of "free sex" sway you into doing something that is meaningless and you might regret later. "Free sex" is rarely free. Often, with girls, there are emotional ties and consequences: getting sexually involved can result in your getting involved in a drama with girls that suddenly have expectations about a relationship. Are you ready to deal with a girl who goes psycho about you because you hooked up and had sex and you didn't call her? Are you ready for the expectation that you're supposed to be her boyfriend now? Or, when you don't meet these expectations, can you deal with the fact that she's told all her friends or even your parents because she was so hurt that she is trying to hurt you back?

> Sex, for girls, almost always comes with "S-EXPECTATIONS."

It is a good idea to get to know the girl better first, and make sure you really like her, which includes trusting her. It is very important to know exactly what she might be expecting, if you get sexually involved. Rarely, is sex free of some type of obligation, at least emotionally, when it comes to girls. This is why smart guys say no to "free sex." Also, there are risks of physical consequences, such as STD's and pregnancy, but we'll talk about that later, in Chapter Seven. Learning to know when you are ready for sex, not just going for it if you get lucky, as well as being ready for a relationship, is an important part of becoming more mature as a young man.

Curiosity—Joe's Story

Joe was 16 and had never had a serious girlfriend. When he was in middle school, he was "going with" a couple of girls, but things never

went beyond kissing. After Joe got his driver's license, he got a job at the mall, where he met "Charon." Charon was 16, too, and she was great. Charon worked in the food court and she always gave Joe free drinks. As Joe says: cute, funny, and sweet! Joe started giving Charon rides home after work when they worked on the same day. Charon was happy not to have to bother her parents for a ride, since she didn't have a car, and she appreciated rides home. After a few weeks, they started getting to be better friends. Charon didn't have a boyfriend, and of course, Joe was single, too. Pretty soon, they were a couple. Within a month of going out, Joe started putting the moves on Charon to have sex. Charon was a virgin and she didn't want to go so fast and she didn't want to have sex.

Mainly, Joe was curious about sex. He liked Charon, but he didn't really think of any future with her or anything. He was thinking that he was 16, and he wanted to see what sex was like. Joe pressured Charon into having sex, threatening to break up with her and find someone else to date if she wouldn't have sex with him. Charon really liked Joe, in fact, she told him that she loved him, and she might have been afraid he'd break up with her if she didn't have sex.

At the time, Joe thought pressuring Charon into sex was OK, because he thought that all girls said they didn't want to have sex and they had to be talked into having sex or they would never do it. Also, Joe was very egotistical: he thought that if she had sex with him, she would be so happy and he would be so good, that she would be happy she said yes, even though he knew she didn't want it. It didn't turn out that way, at all.

Charon had sex with Joe, and she cried the whole time: before, during, and after.

Joe got to find out what it was like to have sex, but it wasn't the experience of fireworks and mind-blowing pleasure that he was fantasizing about. In fact, while it was exciting for a few seconds from a physical standpoint, Joe felt very bad that Charon was in

Why Guys Think They Want Sex—or Not

physical pain and emotionally very upset to tears the whole time, but he rationalized his concerns by thinking, "that is just how losing your virginity is supposed to be," to convince himself that it was really OK. Joe was very sexually inexperienced and he had no idea how to physically have sexual intercourse with a girl, especially a virgin, and he was under the belief that "you just do it."

Charon broke up with Joe after they had sex the first time. She pretty much hated Joe and she gave him the evil eye every time she saw him for the next 2 years of high school. For a while, Joe just ignored Charon and convinced himself that she said "yes," so he didn't do anything wrong. It wasn't until much later, when Joe fell in love and learned how to treat a girl right, that Joe realized what he did and he felt really guilty for being such a fool and so inexperienced and wrong about pressuring Charon to have sex.

In Chapter Eight, we will discuss thoroughly about having sexual intercourse for the first time, without hurting a girl or yourself, emotionally and physically. It is a myth that sex for the first time for girls has to hurt! Sadly, most guys don't know this and as a result a lot of girls DO get hurt. *Most guys really do care and don't want to hurt girls*. For Joe, he was simply curious about sex and he wanted to see what it was like, but he was very misguided about his ideas that girls have to be convinced to have sex and that virgin sex is an event, not a process. Joe didn't realize that sexual relations take preparations and a process of warming up to and preparing for sexual intercourse in order for it to be pleasurable vs. painful, especially if a girl is a virgin. For Joe, having sex too soon, too fast, and without his girlfriend really being ready for sex, left him with having a lot of guilt for a long time. It wasn't until later that he felt so bad about pressuring Charon into sex, just because he was selfish and wanted to see what it was like.

Some girls and guys just have sex because they have heard so much about it, seen so much about it, and thought so much about it that they are dying to find out what it is like. Considering how much our culture talks about sex on TV, in movies, in music videos, and in songs, it is normal to be curious about what sex really is like. This is completely natural and understandable. But, you need to know the truth about sex, starting from the beginning. We will talk about sex drive in Chapter Five: The Beginning of Sex.

As a sex therapist who talks to people about their first sexual experiences every week, I will tell you that almost all women and men are disappointed when they choose to have sex for the first time only because they are curious. A lot of the time, if someone is simply curious about sex, it is not the particular person or sexual partner that is important to him or her, but rather, they have sex as a result of simply deciding that they are ready to try it. Consequently, some people, perhaps most, once they have decided they are ready for sex and want to see what it is like, are not very choosy when it comes to choosing their first sexual partner.

Take a piece of advice: Sex feels different when you have loving feelings toward your partner than when you feel nothing emotional toward him or her. In fact, sometimes this difference is as big as the difference between joy and pain, and between emotional pleasure and physical satisfaction. Just having the physical act of a hand touch you, let alone having more intimate physical touching, will not be very fun the first time, most likely, unless there is an emotional component or you have a partner with whom you can talk freely about sex. The first time you have any level of sexual activity, whether it is kissing or touching or something more, can be embarrassing and awkward, so you need to be with a person who knows and understands you. "Just doing it" doesn't lead to very satisfying sex for most people. Even if the act feels good physically, it can leave you feeling bad about yourself emotionally or simply "empty" inside.

Religion and Sex—Jacob's Story

Jacob decided he wanted to wait until he got married to have sex. He was raised in a conservative church and he went through a abstinence sex education class at church, where he signed a pledge when he was 14 to wait until he got married to have sex, to save his virginity for that special person whom he was going to spend his the rest of his life. Jacob was a really sweet guy and his religious values were very important to him.

When Jacob was 19, he met and fell in love with Rebekah, who was 18. Rebekah went to his church, and she was also religious and committed to abstinence until marriage, too. Jacob and Rebekah met in the Fall, and they kept their vow of commitment to abstinence. After several months, Jacob was finding it very hard to abstain from sex. He felt a powerful sexual drive toward Rebekah and he didn't want to wait any longer. Jacob wanted to get married while they were still in school, in truth, largely because he loved Rebekah and also because he wanted to start to have a sexual relationship and he felt strongly that he had to be married to have sex. During their dating, Rebekah was very strong about not being sexual and in fact, they never did anything more than kiss, on Rebekah's insistence, because she was afraid anything more than kissing would lead to something more and a temptation they could not resist. Yet, Rebekah was in love with Jacob and she agreed to marry. After dating 10 months, they married the summer after they met.

Three years later, Jacob and Rebekah came in for sex therapy because of sexual problems in their marriage. Basically, Jacob wanted to have sex much more often than his wife and in fact, she never wanted

26

to have sex. Not only didn't she desire sex, it hurt when they had sex and she avoided being with her husband all the time. Jacob was very disappointed and also, sexually frustrated. Despite their religious values, they were considering themselves incompatible and even considering divorce. Jacob struggled with the idea of divorce or accepting that he'd have to live a sexless life.

After sex therapy, it was revealed that Rebekah had suppressed all of her sexual drive and thoughts and feelings, to keep her commitment to abstinence. She had been a "good girl" and forced herself to never think a sexual thought or to hide all of her sexual feelings, so she wouldn't be tempted to sin and be sexual. Fortunately, with therapy, she learned to embrace and open up her sexuality, and she developed a desire for sex. For Jacob and Rebekah, their sexual incompatibility was mostly resolved, and their marriage greatly improved. Jacob and Rebekah were very happy that they saved sex for only each other, but because they were so sexually inexperienced, and felt so much guilt over sex, they had to learn about sex, learn to communicate about sex, and realize that being sexually compatible didn't just happen automatically!

Religious guilt is a very serious concern for many teenagers, so it's important to talk about it at length. If you are single, having sexual intercourse before marriage is called fornication, in religious terms, which is believed to be a sin in many religions. Yet, we are wired to be sexual human beings from birth, which we'll discuss in Chapter Five: The Beginning of Sex. We have sexual feelings, but many people are taught not to act on these feelings. Some people are taught that sex is something that God has given us for procreation (to create children), that there can be pleasure from this experience, yet that pleasure is not to be shared until we are married or about to get married. We discover sexual excitement by seeing, touching, and feeling, ourselves and others, yet we are told by those who are concerned for our well-being that sexual activity will be harmful to us. The bottom line is that all of the sexual variations—sex with yourself, sex in marriage, sex with a significant other, or different kinds of sexual interaction—will require a choice you will need to make, and many of you will make that decision based on your religious teachings.

In some ways, some of the religious teachings, such as the value that one must be sexually abstinent until marriage, make life and sexuality easier. Life can be less complicated without the problems and possible consequences of sexual interactions, especially if you are a teenager and single. In short, some religious teachings are simply practical advice to help us avoid making decisions that will harm us. Certainly, some of the negative consequences of first sexual experiences, such as getting emotionally hurt by a partner, having complications with relationships, sexually transmitted diseases (STDs), physical pain, or an unwanted pregnancy, can be avoided simply by staying sexually abstinent, meaning you do not have sexual intercourse at all.

In truth, there is a definite specialness and beauty in being married to, and sharing a life with, someone who has been and will always be your only sexual partner. This makes a marriage of two individuals very special from an emotional and sexual standpoint. However, you should know that, even without that feeling of specialness that comes from being the "only" sexual partners to each other, within any relationship there is still the capacity to create deep love emotionally, sexually, and intimately between two people.

Some religions are very conservative or are called "fundamentalist religions." You may be a part of this type of church or know others who attend these types of churches. For example, someone who attends a fundamentalist church might hear, "You will burn in hell if you have sex before you get married." Very conservative or fundamentalist beliefs are based on control, using guilt, shame, and the belief in a punishing God to get people to follow the church's rules and beliefs. This type of religious training can make people feel badly for having sexual feelings, yet some people believe these teachings are God's law and the absolute truth. The sad part is that absolutely everyone has sexual feelings and thus many people end up feeling badly about sex and about themselves. For many teens, this situation makes normal sexual feelings frightening. For some teens, it makes them feel like they're choosing between God and sex. While many teens may successfully put down their urges without feeling guilty, others may fail and live with the guilt for the rest of their lives. Often, in such cases, teens feel they are on their own and must find out the truth about love and sex without God.

========

Remember: God invented sex. Search for your truth with God.

========

Ideally, it seems wonderful to wait for marriage to become sexually active, but realistically, the truth is that less than one half of guys wait until they are out of high school to have sex. In fact, 90% of men experience sexual intercourse before marriage. What is important is that, if you have reservations about having sex for religious or spiritual reasons, you need to closely examine these beliefs and act upon them according to what you sense is in your best interest, what is best for you at this point in your life. If you do not feel that you have had your questions answered about what is right for you in the eyes of God, then you need to wait to have sex until it is right for you in order to avoid the resultant guilt. If you are not reasonably sure how you feel about either subject, sex or your religious beliefs, then you may feel guilty or otherwise bad, and this will make having sex a negative experience for you.

Sexually Inexperienced—Collin's Story

Collin was 19 and a sophomore in college when he had his first serious girlfriend, Kelly. She was a good friend to him in high school and they had made out a little bit, but mostly just kissing and some touching—above the waist only. They started seeing each other again when she went to the same college as him, and things got pretty hot and heavy fast.

Collin was embarrassed that he was sexually inexperienced, and he didn't want to make a fool of himself with Kelly, so he decided to do some "research" and learn more about sex. Collin's idea of doing research was to search the Internet and look on free "adult websites" to find out about sex. He also went to the local video store and rented a couple of "adult" DVDs to watch.

Within a few days, everything that Collin knew about sex, well, he learned from pornography. After a very short period of time, he thought he knew it all and was ready to take his newly gained knowledge out for a test drive. Let's just say that Collin's approach to sex was not what Kelly was expecting! Collin had very strange ideas about how Kelly might liked to be touched, especially how fast to go with sexual touch.

Collin's first attempt at sex with Kelly could be summed up like this: he made a complete fool out of himself! In fact, it could have made a great comedy skit on Saturday Night Live. Basically, Collin's insecurity with his sexual knowledge and his method of learning about making love with a young women made for a disastrous experience with sexual inexperience. After that, Collin and Kelly broke up and never did "go all the way."

Given the multi-billion dollar adult film industry, it should not surprise anyone, even a sex therapist, that many men learn what they know about the mechanics and techniques of making love with a woman from porn. Sadly, making love and pornography often have very little in common. And, for most women, their desires, needs, and wants have very little in common with female adult film stars: not to mention that most young women's bodies are real, not surgically altered.

Collin got points for wanting to be a good lover. His fear of failure and concern over sexual performance is common. At least he was trying to overcome his fear of sexual experience by educating himself. Real sex education is important, but real experience that teaches through sexual communication between two partners that genuinely care and use their sexual voices, will be a much more powerful learning tool.

Everyone is sexually inexperienced when they are a virgin, and that is how it is expected to be. It is not a federal crime. It can be very sweet and endearing (and fun!) to explore your sexuality with someone loving and understanding of your sexual inexperience. Actually, some people are very inexperienced and unsure of themselves with sex, even if they have had multiple sexual experiences. For one thing, everyone is different when it comes to sexual likes and dislikes. Every couple needs fresh, new exploration with each other in order to discover their own special way of making love together as the relationship evolves, and that's the fun part! Even couples who have been together for years find that a single sexual encounter can involve discovering something new about their lover, or what that person wants on that one particular day. In fact, sexuality is something that can continue to be new and different over the course of your entire life. It is much more exciting to explore this with someone special, with someone to whom you are attracted, someone you can sexually communicate and with whom you are in love.

My Best Friend Hooked Me Up—Tom's Story

Tom was 14 when he first had sex. He was like a lot of young guys, who took the first opportunity for sex that presented itself, even though he "knew better." He was at a party with about 15 or 20 other people, at a girl's house, "Gina," whose parents were out of town. At the end of the night, everyone left except Tom and his best friend, "Jeff." Jeff told Tom that Gina was interested in him and he should "go for it," with her. Jeff told Tom that Gina was in "no way" a virgin and she really liked him and if he talked to her, Tom could probably have sex with her. Jeff knew, because he'd already had sex with Gina the night before!

Tom was really a nice guy and hadn't ever taken advantage of a girl or situation, but he did like Gina and his parents were also out of town and he didn't have to be home, either. Plus, his best friend was setting him up for maybe a sure thing. So, Tom started talking to Gina and in fact, they got along really well. Jeff went home, giving Gina and Tom the "thumbs up" sign and left them alone for the night.

Tom had been raised to be respectful to girls and to always have permission from girls to do anything with them, even kissing. His parent's had taught him to wait for sex until he was "in love" and it was "special" and to always be responsible about sex, which meant to use a condom and protect himself and his partner from STDs and pregnancy. However, Tom was curious about sex, and despite his parent's teachings to wait to have sex, maybe not until he was married, but until he was older, Tom wanted to be with Gina.

Gina and Tom ended up spending the night together and having sex for the first time, consensually. Tom thought everything was OK, until the next week. The bad thing was that Jeff ended up getting jealous, even though he had set them up and given them the "it's OK" thumbs-up sign. Jeff had been drinking and "knowing his best friend," he thought he would never end up having sex with Gina! Jeff got mad and he got a big mouth. Jeff told his brother, who told Tom's older brother the whole story, including the fact that Tom had lost his virginity to Gina. What was worse was that Tom's brother had an even bigger mouth than Jeff and he told everyone, including people who went to Tom's high school. By the end of the week, after Tom had been with Gina, everyone knew.

Things got worse at school. Tom was popular and a lot of girls had their eye on him. Sadly, after the story went around, NONE of the girls wanted to be with him anymore and had lost respect for him.

Then, Tom's older sister, a senior at his high school, found out and she went right up to him at school, in front of everyone and everyone watching, and slapped him across the face, telling him she didn't respect him! His sister loved her younger brother very much and she didn't respect him for having sex so young and with someone he hardly knew. Anyone in the school who didn't know, knew then.

Of course, his parents found out, which was the worst part. Tom said his parents were disappointed and angry, although they were kind of caring, too. His mom was crying and then got mad that he didn't wait until he was with someone he really loved and it was "special" for him. She asked him questions like, "Did you use a condom?" "Did you think about AIDS?"; "What if she got pregnant?"; "Was she too drunk to know what she was doing?"; "How do you know if it was really OK with her?"; "Is this the kind of thing that you will be proud of telling another girl, who you really love, when

Why Guys Think They Want Sex—or Not

you care about what she thinks?" His Dad was quiet, which bothered Tom even more, but at the end of his mom's tirade of questions, he said "it couldn't have been that special if you went for sloppy seconds after Jeff." Tom felt stung by the "seconds" comment, but he knew his Dad was right.

The biggest regret for Tom was that he ended up being disappointed in himself. He was sorry that he was impulsive and went along with the alcohol and the passion of the moment, despite his very own feelings of wanting to wait to have sex until it was at least, "with someone special." While he didn't feel like he took advantage of Gina, and she never felt that way either, living down a reputation of being a "dog" and just hooking up with her, and his best friend doing the same thing in the same weekend, made him feel bad about himself.

Parents teach you about sex because they love you and want you to be happy and healthy. When parents take the time and energy to teach you about love, sex, relationships, and intimacy, it is because they care about you and want you to avoid getting hurt from relationships and sex. While Tom's parents had talked to him about sex, he still made his own mistake. He wanted to share his story, to tell guys to at least think about their parent's values, because it might help you from having a lot of pain and suffering. For Tom, he felt pretty bad about the whole situation, and he ended up staying away from any serious relationships with girls until after high school. It took him a while to live down his "dog" reputation. Tom did live it down, though, by just being friends with girls for a while.

Unfortunately, many parents are too afraid or embarrassed about sex and relationships themselves to provide complete information to you. Another reason that parents don't talk to kids about sex is that they don't want to give kids "permission to have sex," simply by talking about it. Some parents think that if they talk to you about sex or help you get birth control, then they are telling you it's OK to have sex, when in fact, they want you to wait until you are older or married. Sometimes, as a teenager, *you* too are embarrassed to talk to your parents about these subjects, or you just can't talk to them about anything, period. As well intended as parents may be, few parents have the kind of truly open communication with their children that would let them talk to their teenagers about sexual relationships. If you do, consider yourself lucky and take the time to tell your parents how much you appreciate them for being there for you. Giving appreciation is one way to show your parents your maturity.

Realize that your parents are already communicating to you about relationships and sex, and they have been for years. This is true whether they are talking to you directly about the subject or not. Every single guy reading this book knows their parents well enough to know the extent to which they can talk to their parents about girlfriends, relationships, and sexuality, which is often, *not at ALL!* Most of you know how your parents react to sexual topics. If you're not sure, take the following mini-parent quiz. How approachable are your parents when it comes to sex?

The Parent Test

You are 15. You can't drive and you don't have any money. You are getting very serious with your girlfriend and you think/hope that you might start having sex . . . soon! Can you ask your parents to take you to the health department (for free) or to the drug store, to get some condoms?

Answers:

1. Yes; either my mom or dad (or step-parents, grandparents or guardians) would be happy to know I am being responsible about my sexuality and they would take me to a store as readily as if I needed any health product.

Why Guys Think They Want Sex—or Not

2. Yes; I could ask my mom or dad, etc . . . They wouldn't be happy and I would see it in their eyes, but they always said to come to me if I needed to get protection.

3. No; they talked to me about sex and told me to use condoms if I had sex, but in reality, they would be mad or disappointed about me having sex.

4. No; I know how they feel about sex, and they don't think teens have sex, or should have sex, especially me, their son, and I can't let them know I'm sexually active.

5. No; we have never talked about sex. They think that I will be a virgin until I'm married. If I ever brought up sex, I would be grounded for weeks, if I were still alive after the word "condom" was spoken.

6. My parents don't know what sex is. I don't even think they have sex: If they did I can count how many times by the number of my siblings.

Guide: If your relationship with your parents falls in category one or two, you should talk to your parents about sex. They are approachable. You are one of the few members of the lucky sperm club to have parents with whom you can talk, and they will likely be glad to support you. If you fall into category 3, 4, 5, or 6, you KNOW you need to keep your mouth shut, or life will turn ugly. Don't feel bad; my unscientific poll shows that 95% of teens fall into the last four categories.

Am I right? Most parents would NOT be supportive of helping you get condoms, even if they say you can talk to them about sex. Even then, they would ask you a million questions about what you were doing: You would get a lecture about what you thought you might be doing, or have done, and with whom, and where and when, and why. Right?

Parents give you messages about sex from birth. These messages can range from how affectionate your parents are with each other, or with their boyfriends or girlfriends (or lack of them), to their affection with you (are they "touchy-feely" or not?), to what they tell you or don't tell you about dating, chatting online, and premarital sex. Most teens hear these messages *loud and clear* and know what the message is without any guessing. More often than not, like values about many other things in life, these values may clash or conflict with your own mind, body, and feelings. However, sometimes messages about dating, relationships, and sex come *after* you have already had sexual encounters, and then you tend to feel badly about yourself because it is too late to follow your parents' values.

Five Tips on Parents and Sex

- **Do** listen closely to your parents' messages and values about sex, if for no other reason than they *do* have your best interests at heart in guiding you in life.

- **Do** know that, frequently, even if you have problems with your parents, and even if you don't agree with a thing they say now, you will probably understand them and might even agree with their values by the time you are 25. Sometimes, this means that if you rebel against their values, you may regret it later.

- **Don't** hate yourself because you make your own decisions about sex and relationships. Be discrete (read: keep your mouth shut), be careful, be responsible. Most parents will respect you if you act responsibly (with anything, but especially with sex). At least protect you and your girlfriend from pregnancy and STDs with birth control or condoms.

- **Do** know that sometimes your parents will not be able to be there for you when it comes to sex. A difference in values does not mean they don't love you.

Why Guys Think They Want Sex—or Not

- **Don't** assume automatically that your parents will reject you when it comes to sex. Test the waters by bringing up sexual topics that are NOT about you and see how they react.

WHAT TO DO WHEN YOU OR YOUR GIRLFRIEND IS NOT READY FOR SEX

If you don't want to have sexual intercourse, you have a few *real* options:

1. You can have relationships that do not involve sex at all. Speak up about what you want and don't want. It makes you more of a man, not less of one to stand by your values.

2. You can do other fun things besides sex, like hang out with friends, play sports, work, and share other interests.

3. You can have a fun, loving, close physical relationship with someone without having sexual intercourse. You can share affection by kissing, hugging, and touching.

4. You can share creative sexual touch without having sexual intercourse, and by definition, remain a virgin. "Outercourse" sex can be *great* (see Chapter Six)!

5. You can have sex with someone you love: just you. This is called masturbation, which carries some negative connotations in this culture sometimes, but it is perfectly natural and will help you explore your own notions of sexuality without the inherent physical, emotional, and psychological dangers that accompany sex with a partner. This will be discussed later in Chapter Six.

TWO

GUYS AND LIES: HOW TO TREAT A GIRL RIGHT

Guys and lies go hand in hand, by reputation, especially when it comes to sex. Girls learn fast that guys tell lies when it comes to relationships and sex, and they learn to distrust boys. Trust comes from making promises and keeping them. Learning to develop trust with girls comes from learning how to treat a girl right. If you want to have friendships and sexual relationships with girls, you will need to be trustworthy and learn how to treat girls right, for yourself and for them. Ultimately, guys who care about themselves want to care about girls who trust them, too. It's called respect. Mutual respect. It's important. Very important.

For most teenagers, friendships and relationships are the most important things in their life. God, family, school, sports or other activities or interests may be very important, but if you are a normal teenage guy, you think about girls and sex *a lot*. For many teens, friendships, having fun, and thinking about hanging out with friends is what you think about every day.

If you are lucky, you probably have at least one best friend, and hopefully a group of friends, to call, hang out with, chat online, or at least talk to at school. Having friends, whether you are a teen or an adult, is *essential*. If you don't have friends, you know you need to take a good look at your life and work to make this happen, whether you are popular or a big geek. Yet, having someone special like you or even love you, or acting on that huge crush you've had since last year, is probably one of the most important things in your life.

A lot of teenage guys are not really into having *relationships*. This is not true of all guys: some guys want to have a relationship, with all the elements included, like phone calls, text messaging, going out, and having a special, exclusive connection with someone. However, a lot of guys just want to hang out with their friends, spend time playing sports, make some money working a part-time job, have a nice car, have fun on the weekends, and they don't really want to be committed to one person. Yet, most of you guys want to have sexual relationships and experiences, too! This creates a conflict, because most girls *do* want to have relationships, especially one special relationship with one special person. Most girls only want to have a sexual relationship when it is a part of an exclusive relationship with one special person. This difference between most girls and guys causes a lot of problems.

The bottom line is this:

Often, most guys are interested in sex first, then maybe a relationship. Often, most girls are interested in a relationship first, then maybe sex.

Generally, girls and guys have very different interests and motivations in getting together. Often, guys are motivated to find a girl who looks great, and then maybe they'll get lucky and have a sexual relationship. Often, a girl's motivation is to find someone to like or even to love them, and maybe they'll get lucky and have a relationship and best friend to share time together, then maybe have a sexual relationship. Because of these very different motivations in getting together, a lot of girls get hurt both emotionally and sexually from relationships. Often, girls read a relationship wrong, thinking a guy really cares about them, when it might be that he is mostly interested in having sex. It is often very difficult for girls to tell if they can really trust a guy to care about them and not just care about having sex with them. When a girl thinks a guy really cares about her, and then she has a physical relationship with him, only to find out that's all he wanted, she feels used and cheap.

Guys, you need to know that for girls, sex isn't a game. Girls really want guys to care about them and they want a connection that is not just sexual. Even if the relationship doesn't work out, even if you get scared about what "it all means," it's very important to let her know that you care and you need to tell her what you are thinking and going through, or you will both get hurt.

Basically, girls and guys often have different sets of expectations, which is a set up for problems and conflicts. When girls don't get their expectations met, they feel guys are full of lies and don't trust them. Guys feel like girls are overly emotional, mean and full of relationship demands, that can be confusing, and they don't trust girls, either. So, learn about what relationships are, how to deal with girls, and learn how to treat a girl right.

GUYS AND LIES

The Player—Kenny's Story

Kenny was a player. He gave guys a bad name, because of how he treated girls and "played them." He knew all the lies and used them. The truth is, he was very good at it and he had a lot of "charisma": that special chemistry that some special people have, and the charm to go with it. Kenny was the kind of guy that could walk into a room

and all the girls would notice and want to talk to him. He was cute, but not that great looking, yet his smile could outshine the moon.

Kenny's secret was that he liked girls, and he liked talking to girls, and he listened to girls, and genuinely enjoyed it! When he was at a party, most of the guys would hang out in a group together, but Kenny would be sitting with the girls, smiling and talking. He'd give the girls a lot of attention. From a young age, even 7 or 8, Kenny was flirting with girls. He was always nice to them: he'd carry their books at school, he's stick up for someone being picked on, he even went to the girls' basketball games in middle school. He'd get the other guys to go and support the girls' teams and they all loved Kenny for it.

Kenny's other secret was that he would never "kiss and tell." Even from middle school, and on to high school, he would have two, three, or even four girlfriends at a time. All the girls liked Kenny, and he would convince them, make them promise, to not talk to their girlfriend about him talking to them or seeing them, so the other girls wouldn't find out or get jealous. When he got a car, at 15, he would see girls at other nearby high schools, so his high school girlfriend wouldn't find out he was seeing someone else, too. Even in his freshman year of high school, he had older girlfriends, who were 17 and 18 years old, and he usually had at least 2 girlfriends at one time. Until he got caught—big time.

By the time Kenny was 17, he was seeing a 20-year-old girl, and still had a girlfriend who was in his senior class in high school. By this time, the girls starting making demands on him and wanting him to make an exclusive commitment with them. So, Kenny became a liar. To the girls, he became a "promiser." He would promise to every girl that they were the only ones, that he would promise to never kiss, hug, or talk with any other girls. Actually, first he became a promiser, then he became a liar.

Kenny would make every girl feel like she was the only one, and he played them all. He would never introduce his girlfriends to his friends or his family, so no one would find out. And, when he was out with his friends, he would still talk to new girls and flirt and try to hook up with them, too! Kenny seemed like a really nice guy and his charm would make girls think that he could be trusted. He was sincerely kind and nice, because he liked girls. But, when the demands got too much, like when the 20-year-old wanted him to move in with her (and he was still in high school!), he would break off the relationship.

Kenny liked the attention. He liked being the center of attention and feeling like he was worshipped like a God from the girls, especially at the beginning of a relationship. The truth was that Kenny never got any attention from his father. His dad was a big military father that was often gone overseas, and when he was home, Kenny could never do anything good enough or right. Inside, Kenny felt inadequate and inferior, and getting attention from girls made him feel better about himself, for a while.

After a while, when the girls started getting mad because he wouldn't return phone calls or tell them where he was, which was usually because he was with another girl, then he'd break off the relationship and move on to the next girl, which was easy for him.

When Kenny was 18, he got caught. In the same exact month, two of his "girlfriends," the 20-year-old and his high school girlfriend, both got pregnant. Of course, his parents found out about it, and each of the girls found out about it, and their parents found out about it. The 20-year-old girl, whom he had just broken up with several weeks earlier, decided to have an abortion. The 18-year-old girlfriend wanted to keep the baby. She had a healthy baby girl, named Hope.

At 19, Kenny became a father. At 19, he had to wake up and realize what a mess he'd made of his life, his girlfriend's life, and worry about his new daughter's life. Kenny wanted Hope in his life, in more ways than one. First, Kenny had to make up with his girlfriend for hurting her and cheating on her and lying to her, over and

over again. He had to work very hard to get her to trust him, even enough to see Hope. Also, he realized he didn't want any guy to treat his daughter like he had treated girls — as a player.

Kenny was definitely the kind of guy that gives the rest of guys a bad name. He had family problems that made him look for love everywhere else but inside himself. While he seemed like the nicest guy to girls when he was with them, behind their backs he cheated and played them. In the long run, his actions caught up to him and he lost all the girls in his life, except one—Hope.

Kenny got help from therapy and learned from his mistakes. But, sadly, Kenny did not stay with the mother of his child. She never trusted him again and never gave him a second chance. She told him, "Once a player, always a player." Sometimes, there are no second chances when it comes to love.

Nowadays, Kenny does one thing right: he never lies to his daughter and he sees Hope on a regular basis and pays child support. In reality, Kenny did know a lot of ways to treat girls right, like how to charm a girl and do "all the right things"—except for telling the truth and being true to one girl. In fact, Kenny was better at talking to girls, while most boys are too scared to talk to girls. Girls are afraid of running into a guy like Kenny, someone who seems to be so nice, but is a big player. Sooner or later, they find out and it will cost you! To help other guys, Kenny contributed some tips in the next section, on how to treat girls right, to help guys avoid making his same mistakes.

Dr. Darcy's Guide On How to Treat a Girl Right

1. Learn How to Talk to Girls

2. Don't Lie . . . The List of Lies

3, Don't Cheat!

1. LEARN HOW TO TALK TO GIRLS

A Case of Shyness—Tim's Story

Tim was a junior in college, 20 years old and he was a virgin. For Tim, the real reason he was a virgin was not really because he was waiting to get married or for religious reasons: it was because he was very shy. He only had about three good guy friends in school, and he didn't have any girl friends. The truth was, he wasn't comfortable talking to people he didn't know very well, outside his small circle of friends and his family. He was always afraid people would ridicule him and make fun of him because he was socially awkward. Tim never "dated" in high school. He never went to a dance or a prom because he didn't know how to dance and he was too afraid to ask anyone to a prom because he might have to dance. Tim had two male friends in high school and they would hang out and play video games and maybe go and play tennis once in a while or watch movies. He wasn't on any sports teams, either, because he wasn't very athletic. Tim was smart, but he didn't speak up much in class and no one knew him very well, except his two guy friends, and they didn't have girlfriends, either.

Tim felt like a big loser.

Tim was growing more afraid of talking to girls, because he

didn't know what to say. Plus, actually, he was afraid a relationship would lead to sex and he was afraid he'd make a fool out of himself because he was so very sexually inexperienced. Tim started getting depressed and worried that he was never going to have a relationship and he would be a virgin all his life, if he didn't do something. His mom noticed he was depressed and made him come to therapy. He vowed he wouldn't talk there either, but he changed his mind.

In therapy, Tim found out that his shyness was something that ran in his family. In fact, he jokes, he thinks it is a miracle his parents even got together, because both of them were shy and they met on a blind date through their mothers' church friends. Obviously, his parents were not the best role models for teaching him how to talk to people or date.

In therapy, Tim found out he needed to take medication to overcome his extreme shyness, because he got so nervous talking to strangers, nevertheless a girl he might like. He broke out into a sweat and lost his voice even thinking about approaching someone. With therapy and medication, Tim learned to calm down his nerves, to talk in individual therapy, and then he went to group therapy to get more comfortable talking to other people.

Besides therapy, Tim was encouraged to get involved in volunteer work (actually pressured by his therapist), to be around more people. Being socially avoidant, Tim chose to work in a pet shelter, for rescued animals. Tim was more comfortable with animals than people. As his therapist, the pet shelter choice for volunteer work didn't seem like the best opportunity to mix with people, but it was a start.

After a few weeks, Tim did meet a few people and he also met Susan, who was 18. Susan loved animals and she was passionate about not killing rescued animals. And, Susan knew how to talk! Within a few more weeks (Tim moved slowly, so be patient here), Susan asked Tim to go out to get coffee. Once Tim knew someone, he could talk to them more openly, and they became a couple after going out a couple more times. Once Tim started going out with Susan,

he opened up and talked and found out he wasn't really a loser: he just didn't know how to talk to girls.

Tim's case of shyness was pretty extreme, yet most guys do feel very intimidated about talking to girls, especially when they like them. Hopefully, you will learn here how to talk to girls without waiting until you're 20 to have a girlfriend!

Most teen guys spend the first half of their life hanging out or playing with guys. Most guys don't know how to make that transition from talking to guys to talking to girls. The truth is, and you guys know this is the truth, is that: guys are guessing! You guys are guessing at what you are supposed to do and say, and how to act!

Embarrassing, isn't it? That talking to girls is so embarrassing, and the thought of reading a book on how to talk to girls is embarrassing, and not talking to any girls is even more embarrassing! What you need to know is that you are really, really not alone, and I'm going to give you some specific tips on how to do it right.

Let's get real! The biggest secret to getting over your embarrassment is learning how to talk, whether it's to girls, guys, teachers, parents, or your first boss.

For guys, communicating is the hard part. Thinking about what you want to say usually isn't tough: your mind is going all the time. It's getting the words out and figuring out how to do it without feeling and looking like a TOTAL COMPLETE IDIOT FOOL THAT EVERYONE WILL MAKE FUN OF—that's the problem.

First, try to be friends with girls. Don't start with planning to hook up or get a girlfriend or get into anything serious: Just start with learning to be friends with girls.

Some guys try short cuts to learning how to talk to girls: Some guys have their friends write a note for them or talk for them. Some guys try fake names on chat lines to grow anonymous courage. Some guys try drinking or smoking weed to get the courage to talk to girls. None of these short cuts is going to help you in the long run. There is absolutely no short cut when it comes to learning how to talk to girls—but there is a secret solution!!

Dr. Darcy's Secret Three Step Solution for Communication

1. Talking and Listening

2. Self Disclosure + Acceptance = Closeness

3. Shameless Practice

Communication is simply about talking and listening. If you haven't noticed yet, most girls like to TALK. All you need to do is listen, to start off. Pay attention. Look directly into her eyes. Smile. Genuinely care: if you can't do that, and you don't care, you're talking to the wrong person. Move on. Try again. Don't worry about what to say, yet. Just listen, nod your head, throw in a "Wow"; "Hmmm"; "Interesting"; "I can't believe it!"; "OK." Smile. Then move to the next step.

Here is an absolutely sure formula to be successful in talking to girls. It works every time or the girl isn't worth your time!

Self disclosure is sharing something personal, accepting is how one responds to it, and closeness will follow.

First, when you are listening, like in step one, when someone tells you something, be *accepting*. For example, let's say you tell your

48

parents about how a teacher treated you unfairly in class and that you're mad. You might not get an "accepting" response. More often a parent might ask: "So, what did YOU do to make them so mad? What did *you* do wrong?" This non-accepting response may make you feel distant (or want to be), instead of feeling close, right?

So, when you're talking to your friends, or to a girl, be *accepting and supportive*. Using the first example, being accepting about the teacher sounds like: "Wow, I can't believe that teacher was so unfair!" or "Yeah, I knew a guy who had that teacher last year and she jerked him around, too!" or "I am so sorry, that sucks!" That is the "accepting" part.

The "self-disclosure" part is that you must share a little bit about yourself. First, start small, such as sharing or talking about your favorite color, car, band, or food. Then, if you feel comfortable and accepted, move on to more personal things, like talking about your last girlfriend, or even family problems. When you know that someone is listening and being accepting, talk about personal things that are important to you. When two people share personal thoughts and secrets and experiences, they become friends and sometimes more.

Shameless practice means you must practice parts A and B over and over and over again. Be shameless. Everyone feels embarrassed about approaching girls or talking, especially if you have a huge crush on them, but the only way to get more comfortable with talking is to do it more and more. Start with friends, even one or two, including guy friends and then girls, but not with your big crush (maybe try to talk to her best friend). EVERYONE FEELS FEAR! Winners feel fear, and do it anyway! Everyone feels self-conscious and feels insecure inside. Just do it!

Competence creates Confidence

The more you shamelessly approach people, talk to people, listen to people, share yourself, accept others, the closer you will feel, the more friends you will make, and the easier it gets. Remember: girls like attention. They like to be noticed. If you simply let yourself come up to girls, talk a little, and listen, you will get better at it, become competent and grow confidence.

One Final "Talk" Tip: All Talk=No Action

Simply: silence is golden. Love and relationships and sex are special because they are shared between only two people. Keep it that way. If you talk, and brag and tell your friends about your sex life or big time messing around details, you will NOT get any more action. You will hurt the girl. Girls and guys, but mostly girls, are very emotionally hurt by people knowing about them having sex or even just being with someone. Besides ruining their reputation, their parents might find out, and then she may never see the light of day again, to see you again, in some cases. If you can't keep your mouth shut, you have no respect for her, and you don't deserve to get any more action. Oh, and by the way, as unfair as it is, you need to know these are the rules:

Bragging Rights

- Girls can brag.
- Guys can't.
- Get over it.

2. DON'T LIE . . . THE LIST OF LIES

So, exactly what counts as a lie? It is painfully true that some of you guys don't seem to understand or accept the simple version of, "It's either the truth or a lie," so I'm going to give you some guidance here. Obviously, you know that if you don't tell the truth when you are looking straight in someone's face, it's a lie. Yet, a lot of guys seem to be able to convince themselves that some lies "don't count." So, here's a list of lies to make this crystal clear. Promise.

List of Lies

Lies of Omission: What they don't know, won't hurt them.

Lies of Exaggeration: "You're the only one I've ever loved and ever will."

Lies of Minimization: "I swear I only did it ONE time."

Lies of Love: "But, I love you!" "Yeah, sure, I love you!"

Lies of Coercion: "You would if you loved me, like I love you!"

Lies of Lies: "I swear I would never lie to you."

Lies of Respect: "I swear I'll respect you tomorrow."

Lies of Superstition: "If I have my fingers crossed, then it's not a lie."

Lies of Order: "You're my first one! Promise!"

Lies of Recantation: "That's not what I said, you got it wrong."

Lies of Time : "You're the only one [read: that is, today]."

Lies, lies, lies . . . they're all lies. There is only one lie you are allowed to tell that will be forgiven, and it is this white lie: When she asks if she looks fat, or if her jeans make her look fat, or if she looks fat in her new bikini: The answer is, "NO!" And, if she is fat, she's knows you're lying, and she'll love you for it. But, that's the only lie that counts!

3. DON'T CHEAT

Cheating is a lot like lying. For some people, it is real obvious what counts as cheating, but for some it's not so clear. The golden rule of "Do unto others as you would have them do to you" might be a good general guideline, but the vast land of rationalizations for "what things mean" begs for more hard and fast rules, when it comes to how to treat a girl right. So . . . here's the cheat sheet on cheating:

Cheat Sheet on Cheating

- Don't have sex with anyone else. For those who need a little further definition: "SEX" means touching someone's sexual parts, which includes breasts, buttocks, genitals, and rubbing through clothing.
- Don't kiss anyone else.
- Don't go out alone with the opposite sex, without inviting your girlfriend and telling her about it first. If you can't tell her what you're doing with another girl, you definitely are probably cheating.
- Don't have sex with someone online or have online relationships: that is still cheating.
- Don't ask anyone else out or give out your number or take a phone number. No "making cheating plans" that "don't count."
- Phone sex with someone else is still cheating.
- Your girlfriend should be your best friend. If you have a girl friend who is important in your life, she should also be your girlfriend's friend, or maybe it's not just a "friend."
- If you want to move on: break up with your girlfriend first or immediately after you cheated. When you cross the line, the line is broken. When "just talking" is leading to "hooking up," break up first or as soon as possible, or you'll have a bad rep as a cheating lying dog.

- Expect your cheating WILL be found out. Ninety percent of cheaters are discovered—leaving a 10% escape rate. Bad odds. Expect if you cheat, you'll get caught.

4. BE FUN!!

Welcome to the new millennium: Everyone knows that the concept of "dating" is out-dated and has been replaced by "hanging out." Hanging out usually means you go to friends' houses, she goes to friends' houses, maybe you even go to each other's houses, but you just hang out, watch movies, play video games, and maybe talk. Right? And if you hang out long enough, you might hook up, right?

Sure, you are welcome to go along with what everyone else is doing, and maybe even find out and hang out at the right hang out place, but the truth is, if you want to treat girls right: girls want to have fun!

If you want to really have fun with girls, do something fun! Be creative! Be daring! Do something cool! Be the entertainment! Hey, I'm not a teenager and I'm not your social director here, but here's a few ideas:

If you want to have fun, BE FUN!

- Make a CD mix together, downloading your favorite tunes
- Go out and take funky pictures around the house, neighborhood, or town and make your own photo album
- Go to the beach and surf, swim, or sun
- Try moonbathing, like sunbathing, but under the moon and stars
- Go see an independent or foreign film
- Find a teen dance club and go together
- Go water or snow skiing
- Take your boom box, CD mix, and have a picnic . . . day or night, by candlelight

- Make a collage of your favorite things and post them in your rooms
- Go sledding on a snowy day

Ok . . . maybe none of these things are YOUR things, but figure out what you like to do, what she likes to do and do it. The bottom line is, if you want to have a girl want you, be fun, whether you are 15 or 50.

5. YOUR FRIENDS/HER FRIENDS

If you want to treat a girl right, treat her friends right, and treat her right in front your friends. It's called respect.

A lot of teen relationships get into trouble when it comes to your friends/her friends. Our friends reflect our personal likes/dislikes and having acceptance of our friends is very important, especially for girls. If you don't respect your girlfriend enough to respect her friends, then you shouldn't be with her. She should respect your time with your friends, too. But (and this is a big but), your girlfriend should come first!

Be friends with your girlfriend first.

Yes, go out with the guys, hang out with them, but you, if you want to be in a relationship, have to do something very different than you've ever done before: you've got to think of someone else beside yourself . . . first. If you want to have a girlfriend, you've got to think about her and talk to her about what you are doing, especially when it comes to talking about what is going on with you and your friends.

How this looks: You get home from school. You eat. You turn on the T.V. You start thinking about what to do beside homework. You call your best bud. He comes over. You crash in front of the T.V. You get something to eat. You get something to drink. You chill. You space. You laugh.

Everything is going great, except, you forgot something: Your girlfriend!

So, what do you do?

This is the answer to your question: Call her! Ask her about her friends or her day or school or work or family. Take the time to care and listen and remember: acceptance will bring you closer. Respect means you think about her and how she thinks. You check in with her, you talk to her and ask her how she's doing, to respect her like you would your best friend. It takes time to learn how to be a friend with girls, but being friends with girls should come long before you become more serious with physical relationships, especially sexual relationships.

Also, it is important for you not to be embarrassed about being friends with a girl in front of your guy friends. When you are a teenager, someone in your group of friends is going to be the "first one" to really have a girlfriend. The first time someone breaks off from their guy friends to put their girlfriend first, he is likely to get harassed and teased by their friends. If you're the first, be strong and let your friends know that they need to be your friends and support you. Be courageous and stand up for your feelings (heck, why not brag). Or, if it's one of your friends, be understanding of your friend wanting to be with his girlfriend. Respect your friends' girlfriends and they will learn to respect you. In the long run, you'll be relating to girls better, with your friends, her friends, and girlfriends.

One more thing: Act the same in front of friends toward your girlfriend as you do when you're alone with her.

If you are sweet and attentive and caring around her and then you ignore her and act like you don't care that much about her in front of your friends, this will hurt your girlfriend's feelings. It is a huge deal for girls to feel like you care about them in front of your friends. If you act differently around your friends, she will feel like you are not genuine about your feelings toward her, or maybe you're lying to her about what she means to you. She might even think you are cheating on her because you don't want your friends to know she's your girlfriend. Be respectful toward your girlfriend in front of your friends, be real about your feelings toward her with your guy friends, which will make her feel important in your life.

6. GUYS AND ANGER

One of the most important things in treating girls right is for girls is to feel safe with you. Most guys are taught: "Never hit a girl: you don't know your own strength, so never hit a girl." That is a very good start, to know there is a zero-tolerance to physical violence, but beyond the basics, guys need to know how to treat a girl right when it comes to disagreements, fights, and handling anger.

Girls get scared when guys get mad.

Guys get a bad reputation for the way they handle anger, and one of the biggest reasons that girls don't trust guys is what happens when they get mad. It is a normal human reaction to get mad, but as a teenager, guys have a tendency to get more intense with anger, in a way that can be frightening to girls. Yes, girls get angry, too, but most guys aren't scared by it, right?

Girls need to know they are always safe with you.

Guys, you can avoid a lot of anger by following the first three tips outlined here: Learn to talk to girls, be honest and don't cheat. Beyond the basics, what are you going to do when you get jealous or get in a fight?

How to Handle Anger

- No name calling or swearing or yelling. If someone yells, take a break and get back together after you calm down: take a time out if you need it
- Don't punch or hit something in front of a girl, like putting a hole in the wall
- Learn to calm yourself down: try exercise, music, TV, a cold shower, sleep, talking to a friend, driving around, or go outside and scream it out
- Learn to communicate: See #1: How to Talk to Girls
- Learn to listen when she's mad, the whole way through, instead of just reacting to her anger or trying to yell to get her to calm down
- The quieter you get when she's mad, the quieter she'll get
- Admit you are wrong—even if your fault is a small part of the problem
- Say you're sorry—even if it is a small part of the problem
- Make compromises or take turns to solve a problem
- Be consistent and predictable. Don't explode. If you're afraid you're going to blow up, take a time out and calm yourself down
- Let her know you can handle your anger!

> One of the most important things when it comes to relationships and sex is trust.

Trust includes being able to predict how someone might act in a situation, especially when there are fights and anger. Trust means that you treat someone decently, even if one of you is angry. Trust requires that if you are wrong, then you admit it and you say you're sorry.

Sometimes, even if you think you and your girlfriend are ready for sex, it is important to know you can trust each other first, so that you won't get hurt later by the relationship. When sex enters into a relationship, so does jealousy, which heats up conflict. That is why it's important to learn to handle conflict and anger, as a part of having a more intimate and a sexual relationship. Later in this book, you'll learn ways to avoid getting hurt emotionally by sex, particularly by knowing how you can trust a girl to be nice to you and treat you right. For now, remember: Nice guys finish first and they get seconds.

7. MEET THE PARENTS

You have to meet the parents: it's not a choice, it's a matter of respect. Most teen girls aren't going to be allowed to go out and see you, unless you do meet their parents. Yet, a lot of guys can avoid this by simply meeting a girl out at friends' houses or when she goes out with a group of girls or if she sneaks around and lies and tells her parents she's staying out at a girlfriend's house.

Few girls want to go sneaking around to see their boyfriend. It usually makes them feel ashamed—of you. Unless she is trying to hide you because you're too old for her or have some huge flaws, like you've dropped out of high school, or you're of a different race and her parents don't approve, or you have a reputation as the town drug dealer, and she doesn't want you to meet them, then don't. But, even

58

if all those things are true: meet the parents.

Making a girl sneak around, because you don't have the guts to meet the parent(s) makes you look immature, disrespectful, have no self-esteem, and puts her in a bad position with her family. Be a man: meet her family. Be proud of yourself, no matter who you are. Everyone has some good qualities—if you didn't, why would she be with you? If you are afraid to communicate, go back to step one and learn to communicate better. Sure, there are some psycho parents, especially dads, that are scary to meet, but you can start by meeting them at a shallow level at first. Develop some people skills. Practice with your own family and friends. Have the maturity to meet her parents, especially if you are having a serious relationship with a girl, if you want to treat her right.

Meet the Parents: A Simple Guide

- Show up—on time
- Don't honk the horn, ring the bell
- Don't show up drunk or high
- Clothes count—dress nice and neat (tuck the shirt in)
- Hygiene counts (shower first)
- Talk to develop trust. Talk and listen. Answer their questions
- Don't lie
- Find out something about each parent—their job/hobbies/interests-and ask them about themselves, to show your interest (and to let *them* talk)
- If you come for dinner, bring a "hostess" gift (like flowers, dessert, or ask your mom!)

8. GIRLS AND GIFTS

Gifts are important. Learning to give gifts is an important part of being a boyfriend, and later, a husband. Gifts are a special way to say,

"I like you," "I care about you," "I care about who you are." As her boyfriend, you are in a unique position to know her better than anyone else in the world: her thoughts, her dreams, her goals, her likes and dislikes, and her secret desires (from chocolate to magazines to sex!). Learning to give thoughtful gifts is one of the easiest ways to treat a girl right, get off on the right foot, and show a girl you really care—as well as keep a girlfriend.

A lot of guys have asked me: "What do I get for her? I don't know girls! I don't know anything a girl would want!"

The secret truth is: ANYTHING!

> In the beginning of a relationship, it doesn't matter what you get as a gift for a girl. The most important thing is that you thought about her!

Buying, making, bringing any type of small gift will be long remembered, and you will be remembered as being that sweet, thoughtful guy in her heart.

When my Dad went to pick my mom up for their first date, he brought along two Hershey candy bars: one for her and one for him, to eat together. When he arrived, one of her college roommates came down to the door to meet him. Surprised, he gave my mom and her girlfriend the candy bars. Not only did my mom think he was such a sweet, thoughtful guy, but so did her girlfriend, thinking he brought the candy bar for her! To this day, my Dad will pick up a candy bar for my mom, as a sweet remembrance of their first date!

Buying little gifts, or making little cards is an important way to tell a girl you like her. It might be bringing her favorite candy or food when you hang out to watch T.V., it might be sending her an online e-card. After you go out for a while, consider buying her a small piece of jewelry, such as a bracelet or earrings: it doesn't have to be expensive! You can buy a pair of earrings for $5, but if it matches a top she wears, you will really score points on your thoughtfulness, from noticing what color she was wearing and showing you cared. Jewelry, for girls, makes her feel a special bond with you. If you don't want to be that personal, try some scented lotion or soaps, a tiny stuffed animal, or even a cool keychain. Remember: bring anything, even (free) wildflowers you pick up from the side of the road. What really matters is that you let her know you thought of her when you were away from each other.

Don't forget: Birthdays, Valentine's Day, and Christmas or Hanukah. These are the essential gift giving days. Even if you've only gone out for a couple of weeks and she has a birthday, you can buy a card and small gift. After you've been going out longer, buy a gift that supports some dream or goal she has. If she wants to be a musician, buy her some new sheet music of your favorite song or make her a CD. If she wants to be a writer, get her a pretty journal. If she wants to be a mom: bring birth control!

9. THE THREE RULES OF SEX

Rule #1 Get permission

Rule #2 If a girl says "No": STOP

Rule #3 No pain—EVER

All throughout this book, you will learn the foundation of having relationships, especially sexual relationships. Hopefully, you will learn a lot about sex and girls and treating girls right and how to be safe and responsible when it comes to sex. However, if you don't remember anything else, remember this very short guideline, for now and the rest of your life, on the three most important rules of sex.

Get permission. Make sure you ask, and make sure she says yes. Never assume that it's OK to have sex, unless a girl says yes, even if you've made love together in the past. Yes doesn't count if you use force, you threaten or coerce her emotionally (like, "you'd do it if you love me" or "I'll drop you if you don't have sex with me"), or she is way too drunk or high to consent to sex. You can be charged with rape for not having her sexual consent (she agrees and says yes). Read Chapter Nine on sexual assault and rape to learn more about consent. More importantly, you want to make sure for both of you, especially if you care about her, that sex is OK with her, even if you've had sex before.

If a girl says "No": STOP. At any time that you are having physical contact, whether it is only kissing, or whether you are in the middle of having sex, if a girl says NO, stop. If a girl doesn't want to continue with making out, messing around, or even if she wants to stop just before sex, then you must stop. *For one, if you don't, it is rape, no matter if you've had sex 100 times before or even if you're married.* Even in everyday, normal situations, if a girl is uncomfortable, or maybe she is in pain, or maybe she just wants to change sexual positions, or maybe she's just tired, or maybe she wants to get your attention and kiss you first: if she says no or tells you to stop, then STOP!

> When you stop when she says no or tells you to stop, no matter what the reason, then she will learn to trust you sexually.

No pain—EVER. Sex should not be painful. Sex can be painful and hurt girls, very badly. If a girl is not physically or mentally ready for sex, it can be physically painful. We will discuss in Chapter Eight how to avoid sexual pain, especially when a girl loses her virginity. It is a myth that virgin sex has to hurt. However, even for girls who are not virgins, if they are not physically ready for sex, or are not mentally "in the mood" sex can hurt, and it can cause long term sexual problems, for you, as a couple, and for her. Never have painful sex.

It is true that some people try sexual practices, called sado-masochistic or SM sex, that involve sexual pain that some people enjoy and even find pleasurable. SM requires a *great deal of sexual trust and sexual communication, but it can be dangerous for beginners*. It is definitely NOT recommended that you attempt this type of sexual behavior, especially until you are much more sexually experienced and learn a great deal about it first.

10. HOW TO BREAK UP WITH A GIRL

Rebound — Sammy's Second Time

Sammy met Tracy in summer school, after his senior year in high school. Tracy had just broken up with a boyfriend, who she went out with for 2½ years, the first love of her life. Sammy, who was a good listener, was a good shoulder to cry on. Actually, he became Tracy's rebound relationship. Sammy and Tracy started hanging out together after school. After a week, they went swimming at Sammy's house, and they ended up having sex for the first time. Tracy felt like she made a mistake for having sex with Sammy so shortly after they met. Even still, Sammy was very discrete and didn't tell anyone what had happened, and they ended up doing fun things together, like going swimming in the river, hanging out in coffee shops, and hanging after school with each other.

Sammy started getting scared about getting serious with Tracy. After what happened with Lexie and a couple other girls he trusted and hooked up with for just making out, he felt like he wasn't good at having committed relationships. Remember: he was afraid of being committed and really liking someone again, and falling in love again. But, he kept hanging out with Tracy and they had sex together all the time for a few weeks.

Suddenly, Tracy started saying that Sammy was just a rebound relationship and the rebound was lasting too long. One day, Tracy called Sammy and told him they should go out and talk. She took Sammy out to eat, which turned out to be the restaurant at which her ex worked. When Sammy figured out what was going on, after they got there, she said she thought it would be funny if she'd make her ex-boyfriend jealous, showing off her hot, new boyfriend. Then, her ex-boyfriend walked out to the table in the restaurant and starting crying right there in public. He cried out, "I can't believe you're doing this to me!" Sammy felt very weird, strangely sad, set-up, and uncomfortable!

Everyone in the restaurant was looking at them. After a few minutes, Tracy decided she needed to go and talk to her ex-boyfriend, so she left the table and went into the kitchen after her ex. Sammy, like a gentleman, paid the bill, and left, leaving Tracy at the restaurant with the ex.

The next day, Sammy tried to call Tracy, but she wouldn't answer her phone. Later that day, Sammy broke up with Tracy, over the phone, telling her she was rushing into things too fast and obviously wasn't over her ex. Sammy realized he *was* just a rebound relationship and he told Tracy, "I hope you're happy with your ex and have a good life." Tracy wouldn't answer his phone calls, until a few days later, when she said she was getting back with her ex. They never saw each other again.

Poor Sammy was back to not trusting girls again, and he stayed away from relationships for another year after Tracy.

Sadly, most break-ups happen in anger, and people treat each other badly. I could give you all sorts of great advice on how to treat a girl right and break up the right way, but break-ups rarely end with a hug and a hand shake in the real world. Often, relationships end for good when something bad happens.

Ideally, you should have the decency to break up with someone, especially with someone you loved enough to share a special sexual relationship, *in person*. I mean, you can't blame Sammy for breaking up with Tracy over the phone, after she set him up to make her ex jealous, but it's pretty cold to break up over the phone. On the other hand, it's pretty cruel to do some of the things that people do to each other in relationships, too. When people get hurt, they often want to strike out and hurt someone back.

Eventually, when the initial pain and shock is over, two people who cared enough about each other to be sexually intimate should sit and talk about why they are breaking up with each other. To treat a girl right, if you are doing the breaking up, you should at least have the decency to tell her why. Or she should have the respect to tell you why. Sometimes, when someone loves someone, they feel hurt for many years over "Why?" People deserve to know and it helps them close the door to your relationship and recover from the pain or loss of a relationship, and move on.

The worst thing you can do is just stop calling someone. To stop taking someone's calls and not give a person an explanation is cruel and disrespectful of a love you once shared. If you change your mind, for whatever reason, maybe you like someone else, maybe you just realized you don't love them, maybe you're not comfortable with them, maybe you want to move to Alaska. Whatever it is, it is easier for people to hear the truth, than it is to wonder what happened and wonder for days, or weeks, or even years. As horrible as it may seem to tell someone the truth, it is easier to hear the hard truth than it is to wonder what is wrong with them or wrong with you or what went wrong.

Especially if you shared a sexual relationship or a very close emotional relationship or friendship, be mature enough to face them and tell them what happened: for both of you! At least you will learn something, or not obsess over nothing, when it comes to your future relationships. Breaking up, with mutual respect, is the hard part about treating someone right, but it is the right thing to do for both of you.

Can We Be Friends?

Most people say, when they break up, "let's just be friends," or "but, we'll always be friends, right?" This sounds like a really good way to let someone down easy and a really good way to keep a connection with someone you might still like, as a friend. Fuhgetaboutit. At least, in the beginning. It never works for both people when you first break up. Almost always, when there is a break up, one person likes the other person more or they might still be in love with them. If you break up and you're still talking, the person who is still in like/love will have hope, want to get back together, and the contact in person or by phone will stir up feelings of love, despair, pain, anger, and betrayal. Then, it gets ugly. Sometimes, it gets really ugly. The person in like/love who is now hurt or angry may want to get back together and when they get rejected again they might lash out and want to hurt the person who is trying to "be their friend." Forget about it, for now. When you're broken up, let go. Move on. Don't be pathetic. Spend time with other friends, both of you. When you are both over it, emotionally, and maybe both in new relationships (including new friendships), then maybe you can really be friends. But avoid the fantasy than turns into a horror flick when you try to be friendly, because you can't be friend-like with someone who just rejected their best friend.

THREE

SAME-SEX SEX

Same-sex sex is about having feelings for someone of the same sex, whih can be even more confusing than relationships between girls and guys. At some point in their lifetime, many people have feelings for, attractions to, or experiences with someone of the same sex. This chapter helps you to understand and deal with some of the experiences guys have with same-sex relationships.

Homosexuality is a label that describes sexual attraction for, sexual desire for, or sexual behaviors with a person of one's own sex, but most people use the words "gay" or "queer" to describe male same-sex sexual relationships, so that is what is used in this book. "Lesbian" is a word for a woman who is gay. Throughout this book, sexual partners are often referred to as "girls" or "girlfriends," but please know that *Virgin Sex* refers to a sexual partner of any gender, including someone of the same sex or even a transgendered person, that is, someone who feels like they were born with the wrong sexual parts, which is explained later in this chapter. Same-sex sex is a part of life for 4 to 10% of the population.

Yes, up to one out of ten guys is gay!

Most guys know, from a young age, that they have attractions to the same sex, but it is very confusing and almost always secretive. If you've *never* had attractions to guys, by the time you are a teenage boy, it is unlikely that you are gay. Whether you have had these feelings or not, understanding homosexuality, your own or others, is part of the human sexual experience.

Being Gay—Jimmy's Story

Jimmy thought he might be gay in 5th grade. He realized he was looking at girls, but he also looked at boys and was thinking, "Hey, he's kinda hot, too."

Then he thought, "Uh-oh, I'm attracted to guys."

Jimmy never knew his biological father. When he was 6, his divorced mother got remarried, and had another child: he got a stepfather, an older stepsister, and a new half-sister. Despite the family changes, Jimmy's grandmother was the "matriarch" of the family. That meant she was like the head of the family and everyone listened to her and she was a strong woman. Jimmy's grandfather was the only male figure he had. His grandfather was of that "grand generation of people who were trusting, caring, honest, and always there for you, no matter what." Jimmy spent weekends at his grandparent's house and felt very loved by them. Jimmy felt his grandmother would stick up for him: no matter what, which was very important, when it mattered most, when Jimmy was in high school.

By 14, Jimmy was well aware that he was gay.

Just before Jimmy went to high school, he had a lot of friends that were girls, and he went out with girls, too. One girl he really, really liked was "Korena." They would just talk, make out and have fun together, but they never did anything sexual. Jimmy just didn't have any feelings of wanting sex with her. Korena wanted to have sex with Jimmy and told him so, but he didn't really feel the desire or need to go any further than just kissing and making out. Soon after they were together, Jimmy found out that Korena went out and hooked up with some other guys, even having sex with them, which was shocking to Jimmy. Immediately, Jimmy broke up with her. Korena got mad and they didn't speak to each other for several months. Jimmy was sad, but not too much. They didn't see each other again until they started going to the same high school together. When they starting talking again at school, Jimmy thought they had become friends again. Since he had had a relationship with her, he thought he could trust her. He was wrong.

In his first year of high school, on the first day of sex ed class, no less, a guy named Mark sat down right in front of Jimmy in class. "Gorgeous guy," Jimmy thought, "This is my lucky day!" Jimmy got a huge crush on Mark. Mark was a skater, and Jimmy, at the time dressed kind of different, too, with big jeans and chains. Over several weeks, Jimmy and Mark became friends and hung out together. Jimmy totally fell into this huge, intense crush on Mark that was beyond his control. One day, Jimmy wrote Korena a note, because he thought Korena was still his friend, even though she was going out with other guys. He wrote, "I am so attracted to Mark. I think I might be bisexual."

Then, Korena betrayed Jimmy. Who knows why? Maybe she still liked Jimmy and she was still mad that he didn't want to have sex with her. Maybe she was freaked out by his being bisexual. For whatever sick reasons she had, she took that note from Jimmy and made 100 copies of it and sent one to Mark and passed the copies all around the school—everywhere and anywhere she could literally throw them around the high school.

Jimmy screamed inside, "Evil girl!"

Jimmy was totally betrayed and hurt and embarrassed and scared. He didn't go to school for a while. He stayed at another friend's house during the day, just going to certain classes he knew he had to go to, so maybe his parent's wouldn't find out he was skipping school. When he did go, Jimmy began to get threatened at school. Kids said to him, "You stupid faggot, I'm going to kick your ass." Then, the threatening phone calls began. Friends of Mark called Jimmy at home and threatened to beat him up and hurt him.

Jimmy's parents started to pick up on the threatening phone calls. His mom called the school and asked why her son was being threatened at school. The school resource officer knew what was going on: he made a copy of the letter and sent it to his mom.

Jimmy came home from skipping school to find his mom's car in the driveway, which was a shock, because she should have been at work. He walked in the front door, and into the family room. His mom was sitting on the couch, waiting for him.

Jimmy's mom said to him, "So, you're a faggot?" A long, silent pause deafened the silence. Jimmy was very hurt and scared because he knew his mother was very religious and was strongly against homosexuality. Then she said, "Is there anything else you want to tell me? Jimmy answered, thinking, "Well, I might as well tell her everything," and answered "Yes, I'm not a Christian, either."

Jimmy's silence, a silent admission of his homosexuality, and his declaration that he was not a Christian, started a Holy War inside his family.

Jimmy's mother had converted into being a devout Southern Baptist when she remarried. Prior to that, she had been a hippie and they had been "spiritual," but rarely attended organized church; yet, in the last few years, since the remarriage, his new parents' life revolved around the church. Jimmy knew what the church thought about homosexuality: that it was a sin and that the church would reject him, if they knew about his homosexual attractions. More than that, he knew the church would condemn him even though he didn't feel like he was bad or a sinner. Silent for years, Jimmy decided to openly reject the church, in front of his mother, before they could reject him.

The next two weeks of Jimmy's life were pure hell on Earth. His mother put a lock on the refrigerator and kitchen cabinets, and

Jimmy had very little to eat. His mother, sister, and stepfather ignored him and they were gone all the time—at church, praying for Jimmy to change and be forgiven. His baby sister was turned against him and told not to speak to him anymore. Jimmy was isolated and rejected by his family. He was left at home, and he was hungry and starving, except for a few cans of SpaghettiOs. A skinny kid to begin with, Jimmy lost 20 pounds in two weeks.

The phone was locked as well. All the phone cables were pulled out of the wall. Jimmy couldn't call out for help, even to his grandmother. Weak and very skinny, Jimmy decided to leave home. He went to school, he cleared out his locker, and walked several miles in blistering southern heat, to his grandmother's house on the other side of town.

Jimmy's grandmother saw him, looking like a skeleton, and burst out into tears. He had never seen her cry before. He told her the whole story. She told him she would take care of him and love him, no matter what.

Jimmy's mom called his grandmother, when she found that Jimmy didn't come home from school that day. Grandma told mom, with the shock and anger of seeing her grandson torn to pieces from walking so many miles, and rail thin from not eating, "Possession is nine tenths of the law . . . he's staying here!" Mom replied, "Good, you keep him. We don't want him. We don't want to have anything to do with him. He can't talk to his sister or have anything to do with this family anymore." Jimmy was so hurt that his mother rejected him and didn't want him anymore, just because he was gay.

Jimmy's grandmother filed for legal custody of Jimmy. His mother fought the legal battle to keep legal custody of him, seemingly just to be spiteful and hateful, and falsely show she was his loving "mother," but his grandmother won after the court found out the whole, true story.

Jimmy started his life over. He went to a new public high school, openly as a gay guy, and, sadly, he was again rejected and taunted.

Once, he was badly beaten, suffering 2 black eyes, a broken nose, and a chipped tooth. After that, his grandmother paid for him to transfer to a small, but private high school, where he finally was accepted for who he was. During these years, Jimmy made many new friends, with girls and guys, and even began a relationship with a young man. Today, Jimmy is 19 and very happy with his life and friends, living openly as a young gay man.

> Jimmy's advice for gay teens: Be honest with yourself. Sit back and think about who you are, regardless of what other people think.

Jimmy's story is very sad, especially the rejection from his mother and family. He was condemned, starved, beaten, harassed, and abandoned by every one except his grandmother. Sadly, many young gay men have had similar experiences, which is why most gay teenagers keep the truth of their sexual orientation a secret.

Life can be very hard for teens, and when it comes to sex and relationships, it can be even more confusing and difficult. Add in confusion over one's sexual orientation, and life can seem unbearable. The truth is that gay teens are at a higher risk for depression, anxiety, and even a higher rate of suicide. This chapter gives teens some guidance about how to know if you're gay and what you can do about it, when it comes to relationships and dealing with your family and your community.

HOW DO I KNOW IF I AM GAY OR BISEXUAL?

Knowing "for sure" if you are gay can be very confusing. Some people "know" they are gay from a very young age, because they have always and almost exclusively had attractions to members of their same sex. For many people, figuring out your sexual orientation is a process of discovery, with much uncertainty along the path. Generally, a person who is gay is attracted to members of the same sex and desires or has sexual experiences with someone of the same sex. Generally, a person who is bisexual is sexually attracted and interested in having sexual relationships with girls and guys. However, *many people* have occasional attractions or sexual fantasies or sexual experiences with members of the same sex when they do not identify themselves as gay or bisexual. In fact, it is estimated that 20 percent of men have a same-sex sexual experience in their lives, but it certainly doesn't mean that they are gay.

Being gay or bisexual is not a black-or-white situation. An attraction to the same sex may include feeling in love with someone, having fantasies about them, feeling sexual desire for them, or sharing sexual behavior with them. Attraction works like a scale on a number line:

Heterosexual ——————————— Homosexual

$$1 \quad 2 \quad 3 \quad 4 \quad 5 \quad 6$$

When a person is asked, on a scale from 1 to 6, "Do you see yourself as heterosexual or homosexual, including having love, fantasies, desires, or sexual behaviors?" about 90% of people see themselves as a 2, 3, 4, or 5. The minority of people see themselves as *exclusively or only heterosexual or homosexual*, in their thoughts, feelings, and behaviors. For example, a guy who sees himself as a "2" might only be attracted to girls and fantasize about having sexual experiences with girls, but he might have had an sexual experience with another boy of "jerking off" in front of each other when they had been drinking and acting crazy, but he's embarrassed and doesn't want to do it again. A guy who sees himself as a 5 may only be attracted to guys, and identify himself as gay, but he may have had a sexual experience with a girl once or twice, but he doesn't desire to do it again. Many people have sexual fantasies, sexual desires, or attractions to members of the same sex, but they may never act on them or want to act on them with sexual behaviors. Being attracted to or having an occasional fantasy about someone of the same sex does not mean you want to have a sexual experience with them or that you are gay. Most heterosexual or straight guys would rate themselves as a 1 or 2. Most gay guys would rate themselves as a 5 or 6. Most bisexuals would rate themselves as a 3 or 4, or differently, depending on with whom they are involved at the time.

Being gay is more than just having a sexual experience with another person of the same sex. It means being connected to another person of the same sex physically, spiritually, and emotionally. When this happens, the experience tells a person who they are and what they are. Many people find that having a romantic, fun, or sexual experience with a person tells them a lot about who they are. If you are confused about feelings toward another guy, especially if you have acted on those feelings sexually, give yourself this little test:

The Mini Gay Quiz

After you've been out, on a date, or spending time with a guy you think you might like to be with:

- How did you feel with this person?
- Was it exciting?
- Was it "all that?"

For gay people who have heterosexual experiences (and for straight people who have gay experiences), the emotional and/or sexual feeling regarding the experience may be one of big disappointment or "flatness," from an overall lack of excitement with the experience. Then, when gay guys have a homosexual experience, not necessarily sexual, but just hanging out, talking, dating, spending time together, or even having kissing or touching, they feel much more turned on, much more excited, much more understanding of why people even *want* to have intimate, even romantic, and sexual experiences. In other words, this particular version of sexual experience "does it for them."

> Ask yourself, do you feel: "This is it! This is what I like! This is who I am."

Whether you are gay or straight, also remember the types of feelings you have, both emotionally and physically, will depend on your attraction to an *individual*. Sometimes people have initial dating and sexual experiences with someone to whom they have a weak attraction. Or maybe there is a strong physical attraction, but the person hasn't been very nice to you or treated you badly in some way. Or maybe you are not very physically attracted to the person, but you just love their personality and you are drawn to that person for that reason alone. The degree of physical attraction and emotional attraction (or repulsion) will have a big effect on how much you like dating, sharing activities, kissing, touching, and having sexual experiences with this particular person. However, if you feel like "This is it!" and have a strong emotional and physical attraction to a guy when you're a guy, you are having homosexual feelings and you might be gay.

Sometimes people are attracted to someone simply because of their personality or general spirit, not because of their gender or their genital parts. This may only happen once in a lifetime, and people wonder, "Does this mean I'm gay?" If you get into a sexual relationship with the person, literally, it does mean you have had a gay or bisexual experience. But many "gay" people don't feel "gay" as if the experience were utterly different from feeling non-gay: they just happened to fall in love with a person of the same sex. It happens, and it can be confusing when this happens. Some people have the courage to express and enjoy the love they have found in their lives; some people don't. I just say to such a confused client, "If you can love men and women, you can . . . if you can't, you can't." Those people who can love both men and women may identify themselves as bisexual, but some don't. Sometimes they just consider a certain experience an isolated event and don't try to label themselves at all. As stated above, many people have sexual experiences at least once with a member of the gender outside their usual choice, with both men and women.

Sometimes, there is no explanation to when and for whom we feel love or to whom we feel attracted. You can't help who the person happens to be to whom you are attracted: it just happens and the feelings are involuntary. Sometimes it means you are gay, and sometimes it doesn't. Of course, if you are always attracted to people who are bad for you, like people who beat on you, physically or emotionally, or to people who are alcoholics, it is time to see a counselor or therapist and work on this problem, to figure out why you are attracted to people who hurt you rather than to someone who gives you joy. You do not need to see a therapist just because you are attracted to someone of the same sex. Most therapists and researchers agree that therapy can't change your sexual orientation. Yet, therapy might help you deal with your problems with family, friends, and society accepting you, or indeed it might help you accept yourself and the attraction you are feeling.

Silky's Story

Silky's first experience with a boy was when he was 10. It wasn't sexual—it was emotional. His brother had a friend spend the night, named "Len" who happened to be a year younger than Silky. Silky

thought Len was cute, which was kind of a strange thought, because he was a guy. Silky's dad was a single dad and dated women, so he knew that guys dated girls and all that, but for some strange reason, he felt a chemistry with Len, a boy. Due to a lack of space, Len spent the night in Silky's bed. Once the lights went out and the door was closed and the silence of the night filled the house, Silky and Len cuddled with each other. It was a gradual move to cuddling, at first. Silky moved in, then Len moved in, then Silky moved closer, then Len moved closer and pretty soon, they were touching bodies, in their boxers and t-shirts, and they were holding each other. Silky felt that chemistry even stronger. They had a connection, both of them, it was mutual, and Len felt it too. They hugged and cuddled all night. It felt natural. It felt right. They had several sleepovers after that and spent the night together in one bed. Silky wondered what that meant, he wondered if he was gay, but he never talked about it with Len—or anyone else for that matter. He knew enough to keep it a secret.

Silky's dad owned a building company. Dad had several trucks and sites and storage units and he was always working. He told his son: "Boys don't cry. Boys don't have emotions. Men watch football. Men have rough hands."

Silky said nothing and he became quiet. He was very confused. He didn't know what he was going to do about being a boy and liking boys. Of course, he never told anyone. Ever.

Silky got his nickname from his stepmother. Silky worked odd jobs, then at fast food restaurants (everyone has to do their 'fast food sentence' to appreciate life), and he made a little of his own money. He bought his own clothes, and even his own socks and underwear. He didn't like "whitey tidies." He liked silky, fancier underwear. His step-mom knew it, she didn't reject him for it, and she affectionately called him "Silky."

Silky got his first boyfriend at 16. It was a much older guy, who was 26, "Lee." He was the manager at the restaurant Silky worked. Lee had been married and had just separated from his wife. Lee and

77

Same-Sex Sex

Silky worked together and got along very well, and began to talk and bond with each other, closer than the other people who worked there, by far. They were friends, first. Lee and Silky each had their first gay sexual relationship together. Silky's thoughts were, "Wow, this is cool!" Silky had been with a girl once before, a few times, and it was good, it was OK, but being with a man was very different, and it felt totally right. It was fun! For several months, they got even closer, and Silky kind of saw him as a mentor, a successful business-man, whom he looked up to and could learn from, and love.

After 6 months, Lee started acting like a real jerk. He had money and Silky didn't. Lee would joke that he wanted Silky to be his "house boy-toy" and he'd take care of him. Then he would say things like, "I'll take you out for dinner, if you'll put out." Silky didn't like being treated like that. It made him feel cheap and used.

Then, Lee announced to Silky that he wanted to go the big Gay Olympic Games in Atlanta, which was a "mini-olympics" for gay athletes. Lee said he wanted to cruise around and "see what was out there." Silky thought this was one of Lee's sick mental games to evoke jealousy and test his love for him. Lee ended up going to Atlanta, and he cheated on Silky with an older guy who promised to take him traveling around the world—a world in which a high school kid couldn't compete.

Silky was crushed. Lee was his friend, his boyfriend, and he meant everything to Silky. Silky felt like he was older than 16, and he understood he couldn't be everything a 26 year old man could be or maybe even . . . want. They broke up and Silky was devastated, for a while. His first love broke his heart and cheated on him. Yet, he always held a special place in his heart for Lee, like all people do, gay or straight, for that first love, that first time, that special place that no one can take away, ever.

SPECIAL ADVICE ON BEING GAY AND HAVING SEX FOR THE FIRST TIME

Sex for the first time, if you think or know you are gay, has a lot of things in common with the first sexual experiences of people who are not gay. For one, attraction is important. Being with someone because you are attracted to them makes love and sexual encounters special. Second, every person has their own personal "conditions" for sexual experiences. As we'll discuss in the next chapter, these conditions may include having a committed and exclusive relationship, being in love, being a certain age, being in a certain environment, or having a deeply trusting partner. Paying attention to your conditions for sex is very important for having positive sexual experiences and relationships. Simply being heterosexual means you do not have to question convention. The hard thing about being gay is that it means redefining your entire sexuality and your relationship with society. As some of you may have already found out, being gay is not generally accepted at home, in your church, at your school, or even among your friends. In fact, in many parts of the world, being gay results in being rejected by virtually everyone, just because you are attracted to someone of the same sex.

SO WHAT IS GAY SEX?

Remember, gay teens and men are people, and they are people who are sexual. Gay sex is about sharing love and sexual pleasure in whatever way two people decide to connect emotionally, physically, and spiritually. Gay men can enjoy romance, companionship, dating, kissing, hugging, touching, caressing, masturbation, mutual masturbation (masturbating each other with hands), oral sex, and anal sex. Gay guys enjoy the same type of sexual pleasuring and variation that any other young man would enjoy, except they enjoy it with another man. Gay men have likes and dislikes with sex, just like straight guys. Most gay guys like oral sex, some don't; some like anal sex, some don't. Contrary to popular belief, not all gay men have nor do they enjoy anal sex. In fact, only 50% of gay men regularly enjoy anal sex. Mostly, gay men want to love and be loved, which is the greatest gift on Earth.

COMING OUT

"Coming out" means letting people know you are gay, bisexual, or transgendered. The decision to come out can be, and in fact is, the subject of entire books, and I encourage you to search out these resources. Often people spend years, alone, contemplating their sexuality and being too scared to talk to anyone about it for fear of being rejected. Rejection is a reality in our society when you are gay. For many gay people, rejection, or the fear of it, makes them feel entirely isolated, and, as mentioned above, often depressed, and sometimes suicidal. You need to have someone to talk to about being gay! Being isolated and feeling you don't belong is no way to go through high school, college, or life.

The first person to come out to is yourself.

First come out to yourself, at least to the extent that you admit to yourself that you are thinking about or are attracted to members of the same sex. Next, you need to find someone with whom to talk. Finding someone to talk to will make a huge difference in your life. Some people are lucky enough to have accepting parents and friends. With my sons, and since they were young boys, as a preface to any discussion about dating I always said, "When you are older, and going out with a girl or a guy . . ." I wanted my sons to feel like it would be OK if they were straight or gay. I really didn't care if they were gay or not, I just wanted them to have the experience of loving and being loved, and I wanted them to be happy. When he was 7, my son told me, "Mom, you don't have to say 'or a guy' anymore, I already know I'm not gay, OK?" Yeah, it was OK, either way.

Many parents, teachers, preachers, and people in society don't feel this way, however. Many people feel homosexuality is a sin. Many people quote the Bible as saying, "Same-sex acts are sinful." However, some gay churches interpret the Bible differently than this or choose to believe that God will love them, no matter whom they love. Of course, this is a big controversy for our society, and the bottom line is that a lot of people reject homosexuality, but not all people do. You need to find someone to talk to who does not reject you for being gay, someone who will talk to you about it. It can be very hard to find such a confidant, or even to have any idea where to look for such a person. Sometimes parents are open to talking to you about your feelings. You probably already know their feelings about homosexuality. You know if your parents or guardians are "gay-friendly" or not.

If your parents or guardians aren't open, you may be able to turn to your friends. You can "test" your parents or friends for their ability to accept or reject you by just talking about someone gay or by discussing a story line in a T.V. show or movie that references homosexuality. Even if there is a positive response, however, you should know that you will be taking a risk in sharing a very private part of yourself: your sexuality. You should know that, although they might generally tolerate homosexuality, they might be freaked out if they know *you* are gay. You should also know that a *lot* of parents and friends *already* know or suspect that you might be gay. In most of these situations, they are afraid to say anything to you in case you aren't gay, because they don't want to hurt your feelings. This means that, sometimes, people are really prepared to talk to you and accept you. Other family members may also be possible candidates for someone to share your feelings with, such as an aunt or uncle, a cousin, or even a grandparent.

If your parents or friends are in no shape to talk to you about your sexuality, you will need to consider coming out to someone else. One option may be a school counselor or teacher. Keep in mind that counselors are required *by law* to maintain the full confidentiality of anything you talk to them about (except for threats to kill yourself or someone else). Teachers do not have to abide by a law of confidentiality, however, and if you absolutely do not know if you can trust them, try a counselor instead. If your school counselor will just not do, you may try your pastor or minister. A minister is also bound by confidentiality and can't tell anyone what you talk about. If you do not attend church, or if you belong to a very conservative church, this may not work either. You might ask your parents to take you to a counselor or therapist.

You can go to a community mental health center for free, and many medical insurance companies will pay all or a portion of the cost for a private therapist. If the counselor is obviously *not* gay-friendly (which most counselors are trained to be), then find another one. Find one with whom you feel comfortable and to whom you can talk about anything. If you can't find anyone in your immediate family or a counselor to talk to, try to find a gay or lesbian group in the community. Most community newspapers have weekly listings for gay support groups or churches. If there is a community college or university in your area, contact general information at the school and most will have a gay or lesbian support group, often called a "GLBT" group, for gay/lesbian/bisexual/transgendered group.

If none of these options work, go to the Internet. There are many resources on the Internet for gays and lesbians, including resources specifically for teenagers. The Internet is a great way to discover yourself and to gain free information, but as with any contact with a new person or organization, you obviously need to be careful that the information is accurate and the intentions of the people on the other end of your communication are trustworthy.

There are also gay and lesbian teen Internet chat rooms to connect with other teens, and often, these resources are a great place to start before even trying to talk to another person face to face. Also, watch out for Internet "predators" on chat lines, sexual predators that look for teens to talk to, meet, or even abuse. Remember, that anyone can "pretend" to be a "gay teen," but it might be a 54-year-old creepy guy! NEVER give anyone your phone number, your real name, your address, and NEVER meet with anyone you have met on the Internet. Also, please remember that the Internet, or your use of it from your home, may not be completely private: every communication is potentially traceable. If you have a concern that someone may be monitoring your Internet use, you may want to use a public library or another public resource. Finally, remember: connecting with someone electronically does not replace having a personal connection with someone in your life who will support you.

TRANSGENDERED TEENS

A transgendered person is one who feels they were "born into the wrong body." Simply, there are girls and boys who feel like their bodies are the wrong gender. For guys, that means they have all the male parts, but inside they feel like they are a girl. Transsexual is a term that is often used interchangeably with transgendered. While most guys are happy to embrace the changes of puberty, from growing hair to growing body parts, a transgendered teen does not have their mind and body in harmony. Most transgendered teens have known from their earliest memories that they are a different gender, from the age of 4 or 5. Being a teenager going through puberty is difficult enough, with your voice changing and hormones raging. For a transgendered teen, puberty is a living nightmare, to have body parts turn into something that is foreign to them from who they feel they are inside. Some transgendered people have sex change operations, where their sexual parts are changed from male to female, but some do not have surgery, and some can not afford the treatment or surgery. Transgendered teens do need to seek out professional help, from a gender dysphoria specialist or sex therapist, as soon as possible.

A Transgendered Teen—Jenny's Story

Jenny, a writer in real life, wanted to write her own story to tell it to you in her own words.

You guys are probably wondering what a girl is doing writing a story in this book aimed at guys. Well, see, I wasn't born a girl. I have been a guy almost my whole life. The fact that I am now in the process of becoming a girl doesn't change the fact that I have knowledge of what it is like to be a guy.

When I was born, in 1954, "men were men" and "women were women," as the saying went. Males did all the guy things—play sports, take shop in school, mess with cars, get in fights, get a job, whatever. Females did all the "girly" things—be a cheerleader, take home economics, shop, look for a husband, get married and have children. A career for a girl? Didn't happen, not very often back then.

But for us guys, it was quite different. We could do anything we wanted. We had no limits.

This is where I realized very young that I was "different." I would rather have stayed home and taken care of the house: no fooling! I knew how to use a washing machine and hang out clothes on a line to dry, sew on a button, wash the dishes, and clean the house: all the "female" things. Part of the reason for this was that my parents said no matter what sex my brother and I were, we needed to know how to do this to take care of ourselves no matter what. And they were right.

But I really enjoyed it a lot. I liked reading a book more than pursuing athletics. I was much more interested in expanding my knowledge than sports. Wearing glasses got me called "Four-Eyes" quite a bit, but I got used to it, even though it hurt. I hated organized sports, and the only time I went out for anything was track—and I turned out to be good at it since I have long legs. I ran the low hurdles and I won a few races, too. But the "in crowd" of athletes decided I was a threat, so they managed to run me off. I never tried to indulge in athletics again after that. I wanted to be a cheerleader, too, but the girls managed to run me off because I was intruding on their "turf."

So here you have a bookworm, who is happy to stay home, or maybe ride his bicycle, or go swimming, which I was also good at. But the other things that had gone on in my life were starting to pile up in my subconscious mind. I just didn't know it.

I had my first sexual encounter of any kind when I was around 5 years old or so. My female cousin and I used to visit this park in the summertime and she would have to take me to the bathroom on occasion. We "explored" on those occasions, probably naturally so. My second sexual encounter, which was with a neighborhood boy a year older, was when I was about 7, maybe 8. He liked to lie on top of me and rub back and forth on my buttocks with his crotch as I would be reading comic books with him in his bedroom on a Sunday afternoon. In some ways, this was natural exploring, I suppose. But even back then, that young, we knew we could not get caught. I found myself liking how he made me feel when he laid on top of me, the same way I felt good when my cousin and I had our encounters.

I was getting very confused, and the fact that I had a disruptive home life didn't help. My father was an alcoholic, severe and full-blown, and my mother was abusive, emotionally and physically. She dominated the house. It was not until many years later that I realized how mentally sick she herself had been. When I would "get in trouble," my mother's preferred method of punishment was with a leather belt. She would take me in the bathroom and order me to lower my pants and sometimes my underwear. She strapped me across bare legs and sometimes buttocks. And it didn't stop until I was a teen. I thought I deserved this kind of treatment since I had obviously been some kind of "bad" boy, and I would accept it without question.

So you see how confused I really was as a teenager. Throw in the onset of puberty with those crazy hormones running around in my body, giving me new thoughts and strange urges that no one told me anything about—well, I was lost. My own father never even taught me how to shave when my "peach fuzz" started growing. I had to teach myself.

I learned about girls from places like Playboy magazine, in the back room of band class. Human biology in the 9th grade scared me half to death. I hated being cast in with the boys. I thought I belonged with the girls. No one was there to help me understand what was going on with me, internally or externally. I was too embarrassed to ask questions, so I just muddled along somehow.

I hardly dated in high school, even though I thought what I really wanted was a girlfriend. I only had two steady girlfriends, once in the 10th grade and then in the 12th. I was an extreme loner, and because I was, eventually people started leaving me alone. I drifted into the wrong crowd, "the hellraisers," in 10th grade. Finally, at least I had some fun doing what I wanted to do, not what was expected or demanded of me.

I was heavily involved in my church youth group during my later teens. One incident I buried so deeply that it was only this last month that I recalled it. Back then, they had "mock weddings," for the boys' church group, or what was called a "womanless" wedding. Part of the wedding included one guy dressing up as a bride. Well, I was chosen as the "bride." They even had a wedding gown. I remember thinking how much I liked being in that gown, that I wouldn't mind being a "bride" for real. But it was such a radical idea that I buried it, my whole conscious mind just said, "No. Not happening. Not for real."

Then, my whole world turned upside down when my father died 3 weeks after I turned 18 and graduated from high school. You know, you think your parents are invincible, and nothing can touch them, right? Guess again. Real life can send earthquake-style shock waves. I still went off to college that fall, because my mother insisted. Once I got into college, I went wild. The restraints were finally off and I could do what I wanted. And I did. I experimented with sex, drugs, and all kinds of things. I couldn't seem to get enough of new experiences. The big thing I discovered was alcohol, which is very ironic, considering how I had felt about my father's drinking. "Never happen to me," I used to say. Well, never say never, I found out. Alcohol was truly "the forbidden fruit," considering I was enrolled at a private Baptist college where possession of one beer would get you expelled from school.

This whole time, I had remained a virgin. I would not end up losing my virginity until I was 23 years old, which from the era I came out of, the radical late 1960s, was highly unusual. My first complete sexual experience turned out not to be a good one at all, since I caught gonorrhea from it. I caught hell from my family doctor over that.

I kept all my feelings about everything buried for a long time under drugs, sex and booze. Finally, I cleaned up my act, and got some help for obvious psychological problems, like being alcoholic and very depressed, at the age of 48. Still, I thought this guy that I was was so screwed up there was no rescuing him. I found out otherwise.

The whole thing hinged on me NOT really being a guy, see.

I was "born in the wrong body." I am a true transsexual, a transgendered person. When I look back at my entire life, there are so many signs that would have been flare-lit tip-offs if I had only had the proper guidance and understanding, starting with my parents. But I didn't have that, so I paid a heavy price, one that hopefully you fellows reading this book won't have to pay.

Jenny's advice for guys: Please think about this. You are at an age where your life can go in whatever direction you want it to. It's completely up to you. Don't let anyone tell you how you ought to feel. You think for yourself, and then dare to follow your heart. It might be very hard, harder than you will ever dream it could be, but the rewards, trust me, will be well worth it. Isn't it worth your peace of mind?

Jenny is a sweet, wonderful person, who was a transgendered teen, at a time when people didn't talk about transsexuals, and there weren't T.V. shows about sex change operations. Jenny, like most transgendered teens, up until the last 10 years, felt like she was the only person in the world that had these very confusing feelings. Unfortunately, Jenny was born "James." James felt strange and became a stranger to even himself, becoming a loner as a teenager. In college, James became a truly a wild child trying to find himself, and later an alcoholic, drinking for several years. It wasn't until he became sober that he realized all along he was covering up the secret truth of himself: that he was a transsexual. James drowned his true self in alcohol, and when he finally made it back to the surface of life, he remembered he was a girl, hiding in a bottle. Today, Jenny, standing tall at over 6 feet, lives her life as she feels she was meant to be: as a woman and happy.

FOUR

HOW DO I KNOW WHEN I'M READY FOR SEX?

Most guys don't really think through the whole "sexual picture" before they have sex, which can cause a lot of problems, some of them for the rest of their life. This chapter will help you think through many important things you need to consider before you have sex, to know if you are really ready for sex. First, read about the most common sexual mistakes guys make and learn how to avoid them. Second, take my "Are you ready for sex quiz?" and make sure you can answer "yes" to every question before you have sex. Third, read through all the different stories and scenarios to picture what kinds of consequences can happen with sex, before you have sex. Think first, act second, if you really want to understand what it takes to become a man. Don't fall into the trap of what most people say about guys: that you only think with "the head on your penis." Think with your mind first, before you act on your sexuality. This is called maturity. If you really want to become a man, think like a man: think responsibly. A mature young man waits until he is ready to have sex. Even if you make a sexual mistake, you can still learn what you need to know for the next time, and for the rest of your life, about really being ready to be a sexual person, a sexual partner, a sexual man.

THE TOP TEN SEXUAL MISTAKES THAT GUYS MAKE

1. Having sex with the first girl who says yes or just anyone
2. Fear of asking about STDs, then not using protection, and getting an STD
3. Unplanned pregnancy: Not using birth control or leaving it up to the girl
4. Cheating: Not realizing that your sexual behavior can hurt someone
5. Worrying more about your sexual performance than sharing and caring
6. Sexual insensitivity: Ignoring a girl's feelings, like when she's attached, but you aren't, or lying to a girl to get sex
7. Bragging: Talking about what you did afterwards to others
8. SEX-pectations: Thinking if you've had sex once, sex is a free ride and you'll do it again (and again and again)
9. Drunken foolery: Like driving drunk, it's a risk
10. Not having full sexual consent: Stops means stop, or it's rape!

Avoid making sexual mistakes by really being ready for sex. For every sexual experience, remember to think first and consider all of the ten quiz questions for being ready. Be ready for you, to avoid making common sexual mistakes!

Dr. Darcy's "Am I Ready for Sex?" Quiz for Guys?

1. Are My "Conditions" for Sex Met?
2. Am I Not Pressured to Have Sex By Anyone (Including Myself)?
3. Am I Certain I Am Not Pressuring or Coercing Someone Into Sex?
4. Do I Really Know Enough About How Sex Works?

5. Can I Handle Having a Relationship with a Girl, Including Possible Rejection?

6. Have I Considered What Would Happen if She Got Pregnant?

7. Am I Ready to Practice Safer Sex and Use Birth Control?

8. Am I Comfortable Enough with My Girlfriend to Talk About Sex?

9. Is It Legal for Me to Have Sex?

10. Would I Still Have Sex if I Weren't Drunk or High?

Before you seriously think about having sex, you must be able to say yes to each and every question! This quiz is not just for virgin sex, for first sex, but for the rest of your life as a sexual person, regardless of your age or sexual situation. Whether you are 14 or 84: be ready for sex, for yourself and your sexual partner! Each of these questions is discussed at length in this chapter to help guys know if they are really ready for sex and/or a sexual relationship.

1. ARE MY "CONDITIONS" FOR SEX MET?

In Chapter One, Jon's story was about a guy who wanted to have sex because he had a golden opportunity to have sexual intercourse with one of the hottest girls in school. Jon was physically attracted to Amber, but he just couldn't physically, sexually "perform." Jon couldn't get an erection because he didn't feel like he should be taking Amber's virginity when he didn't have any emotional feelings for her. Although this may sound really hard for some people to believe because it is about a young man turning down sex with a beautiful girl, this is a *true* story: this guy couldn't "get it up" because he felt like the situation was wrong for him. Jon found out that one of his "conditions" for enjoying sex was that he had to have emotional feelings for someone and he couldn't just be satisfying someone else, or satisfying his own physical urges for that matter.

You have to look at your own values, needs, and feelings to determine what your conditions are for sex. Some people joke and laugh, saying, "Hey, a guy's condition for sex is that she says YES!" While that might be true for some guys, it really is true for most guys that, yes, guys actually do have values and feelings, too. Everyone has different ideas, or what they value, what is important to them when it comes to making love or having sexual experiences with someone. What are yours?

What Are My Conditions for Sex?

- Do I need to be in love with her?
- Does she need to be in love with me?
- Do I need to be "going out" with her for a certain length of time?
- Do I only need to be physically attracted to her?
- Do I need to be in an "exclusive" relationship (meaning that neither of you have other girlfriends or boyfriends)?
- Do I need to have a trusting relationship?
- Is open, comfortable communication important to me?
- Do my partner or I need to be a certain age?
- Do we need to be of the same race or religion?
- Do we need to be engaged or married?
- Does this have to be the person I plan to spend my life with?
- Am I OK with having a "one-night stand" (meaning you have sex one time and never plan on seeing each other again or having a relationship)?
- Am I OK with cheating, if I'm going with someone else?

Make sure your conditions for having sex are met, or you may be angry with yourself later. Sometimes, if people don't meet their conditions for sex, they feel guilty, dirty, shameful, regretful, or even blame their partners and mess up their relationships. For example, if you think your "condition" for sex is only that you want her and love her, and then you have sex together, but she dumps you the next day because she doesn't care about you and then she has sex with your best friend the next week, you are going to get hurt by sex. Think beyond a moment and consider how you might feel or what you want next week or even next month, then make your best sexual decision based on who you really are.

> Sex is for you and your partner. Make sure your values, needs, feelings, and conditions for sexual experiences are met!

2. AM I NOT PRESSURED TO HAVE SEX BY ANYONE (INCLUDING MYSELF)?

Sex for guys is all about pressure: pressure from hormones, pressure from girls, pressure from other guys, pressure from culture, pressure to perform, pressure from yourself to be OK, pressure to be "normal."

Remember the stories of Tyrell and Sammie from Chapter One? Tyrell had sex for the first time with a girl to prove he wasn't a virgin, because he had lied about it to his cousins. Remember, Tyrell said "Hey, don't be afraid to stand up and say, I'm waiting until it means something important to me!" Sammie felt pressured into having sex by his first girlfriend, and she broke up with him when he said no, which broke his heart. Yes, girls do pressure guys for sex for a lot of different reasons and guys feel like they are less of a man if they turn down sex from a willing girl. Believe it or not, some guys get raped by girls even when they say no! Sometimes guys are pressured into having sex because it is what is expected of you: that you're a guy and you're going to want sex and you *should* want to have sex and you *should* have sex, right?

> You have to ask yourself if you are really ready to have sex for you. If you don't ask this question of yourself, sex will be a compromise of who you are, and the effects of this compromise can last for many years.

Sometimes, it is your self who pressures you into sex. You feel like you want to have sex, so you push yourself into doing something you do want, physically, but maybe you are not ready for emotionally. Sex with yourself, or masturbation, is one thing (and we'll talk about that in the Chapter Five), but that doesn't mean you are ready to have sex with a girl! Sometimes you want to have sex, just to "to be a man." Sex won't make you a man: that's an illusion that only puts more pressure on you to be someone or some thing you are not. Becoming a man is a process of growing more mature, not an event of sex!

Sometimes, however, the pressure is from your friends. If a friend puts pressure on you or teases you continually because you are a virgin, then he or she is not your friend. A friend will respect you for who you are, including understanding your values and conditions for sex. Sometimes friends can make *you* put pressure on yourself to lose your virginity, although if you really look at what you want and who you are, you might find *it is you* trying to please your friends rather than doing what you want. *Just being able to say you are no longer a virgin is not going to make you feel any better about yourself than you did when you were a virgin, especially if you have sex in the wrong situation, for the wrong reasons, and with the wrong person. Basically, making a sexual mistake can make you feel a lot worse!*

> You will always remember your first sexual experiences.

You want to be proud when you remember that your first experiences reflected your personal desires, who you are, and your own sense of timing, even *if*, in the long run, *you* decide that you made a mistake when you look back at the circumstances. Most importantly, you need to know in the future that you made the best choice you could with the knowledge you had about yourself, sex, and your partner at the time. At least you can say, "I did it *my way*." You want sex to be special for you, not something you did just to "get it over with" or to prove something to your friends. Really, most good friends secretly wouldn't respect you doing something that you didn't feel was right for yourself anyway. Another truth is that many of those same people who are driving you to have sex secretly regret their first sexual experiences, but they're not likely to tell you because they don't want to admit it to anyone, perhaps not even to themselves.

95

Ask yourself: Are you having sex just to be popular?

Popularity has to do with a lot of different things, depending on your community, your school, and your friends. Feeling good about yourself, what we call self-esteem, is something that you earn—you don't just get it from having sex. In fact, sex can have the opposite effect and leave you feeling the only thing you are liked or known for is sex. Is that really what you want to be known for? Working on finding your natural talents and gifts and using them is what really makes you feel good about yourself.

Self-esteem comes from doing "esteemable acts."

Self-esteem is earned from you being you, and being good at it, not from doing what other people think you should do.

How Do I Know When I'm Ready for Sex?

3. AM I CERTAIN I AM NOT PRESSURING OR COERCING SOMEONE INTO SEX?

Guys have a very bad reputation for pressuring and coercing girls into having sex. Coercion is an emotional way to force someone to do something they don't want to do. The most common way that guys pressure and force girls into having sex is by threatening to break up with them, threatening to not love them or not spend time with them, or tell lies unless they have sex with you. For example, "If you loved me, you'd have sex with me," or "If you won't have sex with me, I'll find someone who will," or "If you don't want to have sex, I'll find better things to do," or "If you don't have sex me, I'll tell everyone you did anyway!" are ways to coerce a girl into having sex. If you have to pressure or coerce a girl to have sex, you are not ready to have sex and she is not ready to have sex. Coercion and pressure hurts girls, and it is wrong!

Some guys think they are supposed to pressure girls into having sex, or it will never happen, so they have to be the strong ones, the sexual initiator, the convincer, the controller of sex. NO! A lot of guys don't understand girl's feelings and they try to override the girl's feelings with their own feelings, their sexual feelings of wanting to have sex. Chapter Eight talks about how to have a sexual relationship with a girl without any type of sexual coercion, involving sexual touch that is only wanted.

> You are not ready for sex until you can understand a girl's feelings. Until you can initiate and ask for sex and know when she says yes she means it, wait to have sex.

Guys and Empathy

First: Learn empathy. Before you are ready for sex, you need to learn the emotional skill of empathy. Empathy means you can understand someone's feelings. A guy needs to first be able to feel a girl's feelings, before he has sex with her. This means that you have got to be able to know if she wants to be with you, if she likes you, if she consents to sex, if you're pressuring her, or if she is scared.

You don't want to hurt another person with your sex.

In order to NOT hurt a girl, you have to be able to have empathy. When you know you can understand where a girl is coming from, then you can move forward to being closer to her. Empathy is an emotional response to another person. It means putting yourselves into the other person's shoes and trying to understand how s/he might feel.

What empathy looks like: You get home from school, sit down on the couch, and put your hands in your head with frustration over a difficult day in class. You just had a heated discussion with your teacher and you are frustrated and mad. Your mom walks into the room and sees your head held low, with your hands covering your face.

NO empathy sounds like: "Oh, GEEZ! What did you do NOW?"

Empathy sounds like: "Hey, are you OK?" followed by giving you full attention and listening without interruption. An empathic statement is: "I am so sorry; this must be so frustrating for you!"

An empathic response is making a statement to someone and reflecting genuine concern about how that person feels, whether you are on target about the exact emotion or not. Using the example above, you may in fact be feeling *hurt*, not *frustrated*, over your bad day at school, but you feel cared for when you are treated with empathy.

Before you are ready for a sexual relationship with a girl, you need to learn to have an emotional relationship. Sex is not just a physical relationship: it includes emotional feelings and an emotional connection, especially for girls. Most girls want an emotional relationship first, then a sexual relationship. So, to have a sexual relationship with girls, you will need to first learn the skill of empathy, in order to be emotionally responsive, sexually attentive, and ready for sex.

4. DO I REALLY KNOW ENOUGH ABOUT HOW SEX WORKS?

Do you really know enough about sex to be ready for sex? Honestly? If you have never had sex before, you are not going to know what you are doing. Before having sex for the first time, take time to learn as much as you can about how sex works, both physically and emotionally, for yourself and your partner. If you are like most guys, you might be very interested and curious and desirous of trying sex, but you are also nervous and scared about what it's *really all about and what to do*. In this section, you will get some beginning guidance to help you take things one step at a time, and in Chapters Six and Eight, more detailed information on sex is discussed. Take time to learn more about sex to be prepared for a sexual relationship, and you will avoid embarrassing yourself and hurting the girl, too.

Secretly, most guys feel embarrassed and nervous about sex and have many questions, just about the basics of how sex works. If you do too, you are not alone!

Secret Virgin Sex Questions Guys Want to Ask

- How do I get her to consent to sex?
- What am I supposed to touch? How? How long?
- Where do I put it in?
- When do I put it in?
- How long is it supposed to last?
- How fast do I go?

- What makes for good sex?

- What about wetness?

- Where are her sexual parts: The hymen? The vagina? The clitoris? The labia(s)?

- How does she have an orgasm?

- What do I do after I finish?

It is a common sexual myth that a guy is supposed to know what to do when it comes to sex and know how to make everything happen. This myth is very unfair and wrong to both boys and girls. A guy can not know what any girl likes and what she doesn't like. It is not a guy's responsibility. It is a girl's responsibility to know her own body, to learn what she likes, and find out how she responds to touch, a particular person, or to sex. Yet, it is a good idea to learn as much as you can about girls, so you can explore and learn together, whether it is kissing, touching, talking, or eventually being sexually active.

To know whether or not you are ready for sex, you will need to know your body and a girl's body well enough to have sex. Many girls think that guys will know more about a girl's body than she will, and many girls depend upon the guy to get them turned on. In reality, only a girl knows what gets them turned on, how to get themselves turned on, and be confident enough to tell a guy what they want or like. If you do not know your own body and a girl's body, you are not physically ready for sex! Most girls do not, in fact, have a "sexual voice" to say what they think and feel when it comes to sex. As a guy, one of the first steps to being a great boyfriend is to help girls by giving them "permission" to talk about how they feel, to speak up about their likes and dislikes, or to have a "sexual voice."

> Encourage a girl to feel comfortable in using her
> sexual voice, by being accepting.

At first, you will not know how you will respond to being with a girl in a physical way, because you can't always predict your response. In your first physical experiences with girls, kissing and touching will be new and you really will not know how you feel until you have this experience. Take time with a girl to experience kissing and touching each other in many ways, or with different partners over time, just to see what you like. You will begin to get an idea about what you like. With most guys, if you like a girl, just about anything will make you feel excited, and get you turned on. Your body will respond in an obvious way to you: you will get an erection. For girls, what turns them on is not as obvious to them, because the biggest sign of sexual arousal is not standing in front of them: it is lubrication of the vagina. Since it is on the inside, some girls don't know and feel their excitement in the same way that you do.

Girls need to have a longer period of sexual exploration, to know their own feelings from kissing and touching. Most of the time this exploration will lead to physical feelings of sexual excitement, for both of you. Yet, girls need to understand and be comfortable with their feelings of sexual excitement, prior to having sexual intercourse. If a girl is not physically aroused before sex, it is very likely that she will feel sexual pain and sex will hurt her and she will not like sex.

Girls need to learn what parts of their body they like to have touched, or not touched, and learn to share this information with you. Your girlfriend may love you very much, but she might expect that you will be a mind reader. You need to encourage her to tell you what she likes, and you will need to tell her what you want, as well.

The following is true for *all girls*: When she is a virgin, she will need to physically prepare herself for intercourse in order to have physical pleasure when you have sex for the first time. This is fully explained in detail in Chapter Eight, on how to have sexual intercourse with minimal or no physical pain. The basic idea is that a girl's vagina needs to be slowly introduced to having penetration with touch long before penetration occurs using an erect penis. So you see, in order to be ready for sex, you have to understand about how a girl works, how sex works and take it one step at a time to be ready for sex.

5. CAN I HANDLE HAVING A RELATIONSHIP WITH A GIRL, INCLUDING POSSIBLE REJECTION?

LOVE HURTS. Or so the song goes, but it is true. Almost all teenage relationships end. When sex is involved, more feelings happen, especially hurt and anger. If you're going to have sex with a girl, it is highly likely that it will involve a relationship, which can have a lot of drama and complications. It can also mean that you might fall in love and she breaks up with you. Can you handle it? Think about it: Are you ready for a relationship, and possibly being rejected, too?

First Love: Falling in Love and Breaking Up—Daniel's Story

(Note: Daniel wanted to tell his story his own words)

> I was 15. Her name was Kara. She had red hair. She was as hot and fiery as her redheaded nature. She didn't seem to like me at first. Of course, I just acted like I didn't notice her. But every time I thought of her—well—let's just say it turned me on, if you know what I mean.
>
> After a football game, when I was in 10th grade, real early in the season, I went to a party after the game. Kara was there. I was shy, really, but I was getting a lot of attention because I had a really good game and I kind of felt like a hot shot, especially after of couple

of beers (which I hardly ever drank—really). I went up to Kara and asked her if she'd seen the game, which of course I knew she had, but I thought it would be a good way to talk to her. Now, it's not like I didn't have friends that were girls because I did; actually, I had two or three really good girl *friends*. I was a good friend, too—I listened to them and they listened to me. But, when it came to talking to Kara, though, I couldn't freaking *talk*—it's like I went mute, like I did an instant Helen Keller right there. I couldn't hear, talk, or see straight. I felt paralyzed in front of her and stupid looking because I couldn't seem to speak, at least more than a few words. I smiled and nodded my head, but really I worried I was going to get an erection in front of her and would be even more embarrassed.

Amazingly, Kara smiled and talked enough for the both of us. We were in the kitchen at this guy's house I knew, and we just stood in there sort of talking, for the longest time. Before the end of the night, we were kissing outside behind the garage. I mean, we were really deep, tongue lashing, pressing together kissing! She was wearing a short khaki skirt and tights and her legs were cold and she pressed up against me. But that's all we did—kiss and hug tightly.

It was an awesome feeling, like electricity, like a connection, that I felt toward her. Heck—maybe it was just lust—but it was awesome! It makes me smile still today to think about it. Yeah—we guys—we do think about it, too, come on, even just that: a kiss, a hug, and holding, not just sex. Kara would be my first. We didn't have sex until after Christmas, on Christmas break that year, after I'd turned 16. She was not a virgin. She was 16, but she'd had a boyfriend before me and had sex with him two times. Me? Heck, I didn't know what I was doing. I wish I could have been a *lot* more confident and thinking about *her*. I was thinking about *me:* what I would do and would I be OK and alright, or just know exactly what to do and where the parts all went together. I mean—it is different knowing and doing it.

Thankfully, Kara was really sweet, although she did laugh at me, too, but that was OK—it made me feel more relaxed to laugh.

We used a condom and that was cool. Mostly, I was just really grateful that she wanted me to have sex with her and YES! I was totally ready. I'd been thinking about it since the day I met her, when I first saw her (I must say with some embarrassment, but it's true).

You'd think I'd just want to jump her, the first day we made out, but really, I didn't, I mean, I really wanted to get to know her for who she was first. I mean, by the 10th grade you know there's girls who are witches and they will treat you bad and cheat. Really, I didn't want to get hurt and get dumped. I didn't. I ended up totally falling in love with her, but not until later. Or, maybe, I was in love with her that first day we made out and I didn't even know it, but I didn't say the "L" word until after we had sex.

We went together around 2 years. Most of the time, it was awesome.

103

I was really heartbroken when she broke up with me. I mean REALLY heartbroken. I was so sad and depressed and I just wanted to die. I would just sit in my room and listen to really depressing music that depressed me even more. That's where my friends really came in, actually, especially my girl friends. They made me get out of my hole, "the cave," and go hang out with them. It helped some. So did my cell phone. I measured my worth by how many missed phone calls I got, at least for a while. As they increased, I felt better, as stupid as that sounds now. Why didn't I bother to call people? I was too depressed.

Then, a couple of months later, she made out and had sex with one of my best friends. Ugh—I felt like, "Just kill me!" Then, I really wanted to die, but I didn't. I just talked to other girls who were really a lot more understanding than guys. I felt embarrassed to talk to most of my guy friends, they didn't seem to get it. They were just like, "Hey, she's a ho, get over it. Go find someone else." Girls understood more.

A few months later, I met another girl and I fell in love again. The point is this: I NEVER thought that I'd ever feel love and sex and a connection like I did with Kara again—never. But, surprisingly, I did! Actually, I fell in love even stronger.

This is the biggest thing I want you guys to know: Even if you're totally in love with a girl and she cheats on you or dumps you, yeah, you're going to feel really, really bad. You might even feel like you want to die, like I did, at least for some moments. Do this: talk about it to your friends. If your guy friends can't relate, talk to girls. And, get back out there! There's a lot of really great, trustworthy girls. You can and will fall in love again. Believe me, there is true love, and you can do even better, as hard as that is to believe!

Daniel's mom made him come in for therapy because he was so depressed, which is how I met him. He thought about dying and he thought about suicide, and he thought about how he might do it, which is very serious. However, he didn't really want to die, he just wanted to stop feeling so hurt and rejected (before he fell in love the second time). Daniel also felt like he would never ever love someone like he loved Kara. Daniel felt like Kara was so special, and the truth was that she was special, but she wasn't the only special person he would ever be with in his life.

When you are going through a really bad break up, it is hard to believe you will ever feel good again. It is also hard to believe that you will ever fall in love again, especially as intensely as the first time. It also feels like no one can understand because most adults tell you that when you're a teenager, it's just "puppy love," and they don't believe it is as strong as love as an adult and it's not important.

Teens can and do fall in love just as strongly as adults do! Actually, sometimes adults go back to their high school reunions many years later, even 40 years later, and find that special person they were in love with and feel the same feelings all over again, and sometimes get back together! If "puppy love" was so insignificant, how could it last 40 years? A lot of your friends who haven't been in love may not understand, either.

Remember this: you can and almost certainly will fall in love again, even if it is hard to believe when your heart and every other part of your body is aching after a break up. In fact, it might be even better and stronger the next time.

> The truth is, if you have a powerful capacity to love, you can and will love again.

If and when you get into a break up situation, try not to be so isolated. Force yourself to get out and be with your friends. Call people on your cell phone contact list, even if you don't talk about the break up. If you don't have any friends, or even if you do, try to talk to your family. Try to find someone in your family—we're talking anyone: parents, sister, brother, stepsiblings, aunts, uncles, or grandparents. Think about anyone in your family who has been through a break up or divorce or someone who cares about you. Most family members do want to listen and help. If you have no one to talk to, go to see a school counselor, a teacher, or go to a therapist, even for a few sessions. Don't do it alone. Being alone is lonely. Guys need someone to talk to, or at the very least, to just hang out with to know someone cares.

Before you consider having a sexual relationship, you need to consider all of the potential emotional consequences of sex and be ready to deal with them. Guys get hurt by sex, just like girls. The biggest one is being emotionally rejected or hurt. The most common ways that guys are emotionally hurt are as follows:

- Being rejected or your girlfriend breaking up with you.
- Sex can also change a relationship in that girls tend to have more expectations for a deeper emotional commitment to a relationship, especially after things get sexual. Some guys want this deepening of the relationship and some don't even know how to do

this. If the two of you want different things, you can get hurt.

- Almost all teenage relationships end. Can you handle the reality of loving and losing love?
- Not having privacy with your girlfriend about sex. This usually means your girlfriend is a big mouth or brags about it and tells everyone what you did.
- This may or may not bother you, but what if your mom or dad found out?

Emotionally, it is very important that you trust your girlfriend to treat you the way you want to be treated. You and your girlfriend need to talk about what sex means to you, before sex. Are you guys just playing around, or do you expect a deeper emotional relationship, and an exclusive sexual relationship? If you find out after sex that you wanted different things, you will feel rejected, hurt, and disappointed. You need to talk about whether or not you feel ready to handle the emotional consequences that sex can bring to a relationship.

SEX-pectations

Sex-pectations for guys usually means that if you are going out with a girl, then you expect you're going to have sex again and again and again, right?

For girls, the expectations are different. Girls expectations are about emotions and how you treat them and how much time you put into the relationship. For many girls, if they are sharing themselves sexually, they also want to share a deeper emotional relationship. Every girl is different, but here are some of the common sexpectations from a girl.

Sex-pectations: Girl Style

- An exclusive commitment to only date each other
- You see each other at school every day

- You hang out together every day or a few days a week
- You definitely spend one weekend night together
- You talk on the phone one or more times a day
- You answer phone calls when she calls
- You text message every day and answer texts that she sends
- You don't have sex with anyone else
- You answer emails
- Your don't talk to other girls one-on-one at length
- You give her gifts
- You meet the parents
- You go to her family parties
- You invite her to your family parties
- You pay for "dates" or going out to eat and movies

Generally, sex-pectations mean a "deeper intimacy," which includes an increase in the expectations of some type of communication or contact between the two of you on a regular basis. You may also want to share your feelings about things more deeply, like your feelings toward each other or your experiences in your past. In most cases, emotionally, girls feel they would like to have an increase in intimacy when there is sex involved in the relationship *and* they expect the relationship to be exclusive.

Can you handle this? Are you ready to talk to a girl every day and have the expectations that you see her and talk to her at school or after school several times a week?

You need to discuss this with your potential girlfriend *before* sex. Second, you must trust the girl to respect your privacy regarding sex. A good sexual partner will be discreet (read: keep her mouth shut) about your personal and sexual relationship. Is your girlfriend a gossip? Is she good at keeping secrets? Or does she have "female secrets" which can mean she tells her best girlfriend it's a secret and to not tell anyone, then her girlfriend tells her other best girlfriend it's a secret and to not tell anyone, and so on, until everyone you know knows. Is she a drama queen and you are the center of her next drama? Can you handle this, just to have sex?

6. HAVE I CONSIDERED WHAT WOULD HAPPEN IF SHE GOT PREGNANT?

One in ten teen girls will get pregnant by the time she is 18. One in five sexually active teens gets pregnant. If you decide to become sexually active, there is a 25% chance that your teenage girlfriend will get pregnant before she is 20. If you do not practice *any* birth control, there is a 90% chance that she will get pregnant within a year of becoming sexually active (Alanguttmacher.org, 2006). One of the strangest things that I saw, when I counseled runaway teenagers, is that very few sexually active teenage girls ever expect that they will get pregnant, even when they aren't using any birth control. Yet, almost none of them *want* to get pregnant. Somehow they just magically think they won't get pregnant. This is called *denial*: not facing the truth. *If you are thinking of becoming sexually active or you are sexually active, one of the most important things that you and your girlfriend need to consider is how you would handle an unexpected pregnancy.*

Unexpected pregnancy is a reality for teens, and as a guy, you have very little control over what happens when the girl gets pregnant.

The following information is a guide to your options in this situation, none of which are easy solutions to a difficult problem. Below are the four different options you need to discuss with your girl friend before you engage in sex. If you only read one part of this book, this may be the most important section to read!

The Four Options for Dealing with an Unexpected Pregnancy

1. She has an abortion: which is totally *her* choice.

2. She has the baby, raises it herself: you pay child support.

3. She has the baby and she makes a plan for its adoption.

4. She has the baby and you get married or live together.

First, as a guy, it is very important for you to know that if your girlfriend or sexual partner gets pregnant, you have very limited control over what happens. In the United States, it is the girl's decision as to how to handle an unplanned pregnancy, her pregnancy. Usually, the first biggest decision for a teenage girl, is whether to have an abortion or continue with the pregnancy. Ultimately, the decision is the girl's decision alone: a guy has absolutely no legal say in whether a girl has an abortion or not. Some people have a problem with this fact, and believe a guy should legally be able to make a girl have an abortion or, in some cases, not to have an abortion. Despite protests from both sides, it is always a girl's choice.

In almost all cases, a guy has no choice over whether or not he will financially support a child that he fathered: almost all guys have to support their children, and almost all guys will be ordered by a judge and court to do so, in the form of "child support" payments. Child support is monthly payments to the mother of your child. Generally, the amount of child support depends on how much money you make. Every state has different "guidelines" or amounts that a guy has to pay toward the support of their children until they are 18 or they finish high school, and even up to the age of finishing college, or forever, if the child has special medical needs. A good rule of thumb for the amount of the payments for one child is approximately 25% to 30% of what you earn. Even if you don't have a job, you will be expected to get one and pay support for your child, or you can go to jail!

A guy does have a legal choice over the decision of adoption. A girl can make a choice to plan for adoption, but the adoption can not take place unless the father signs away his legal parenting rights, or a termination of parental rights. Even if a girl wants to plan for adoption, she can't do it if you will not agree to terminate your legal rights. However, if you've not been supporting the mother during pregnancy or the child, your rights can easily be terminated. See Chapter Seven for more information on rights of unwed fathers.

A guy has a choice of whether or not he chooses to participate in a child's life and whether or not he chooses to be a part of the mother's life, including making a decision about marriage. If you do marry, please read below about teenage marriage. If you do not get married, which is the case for most teenagers, almost all of the time, the girl will get custody of the child, especially for a baby. You will have the right to have visitation with your child. Later, we will discuss having a relationship with the mother of your child. For now, it is important for you to know that it is your choice whether or not or how much you will participate in your child's life.

The reality is that most guys, like girls, do not think about the fact that a girl can and will get pregnant if you are sexually active and do not use birth control each and every time. Also, most teens don't realize that birth control is NEVER 100% effective! Even the very best forms of birth control have very small, but real, failure rates, which will be discussed in Chapter Seven. The reality of pregnancy is brutal and life-changing for most teens, no matter how the two of you or, ultimately she, decides how to handle the pregnancy. The following story illustrates the reality of an unexpected pregnancy, in the oh, so common case that the couple never discussed the possibility of pregnancy before they had sex.

An Unplanned Pregnancy—Dirk's Story

Dirk was 20 and his girlfriend "Eva" was 18 when she found out she was pregnant. Dirk was almost a junior in college and Eva had just graduated from high school, when they started seeing each other. For Dirk, at first, he was just "hooking up" with Eva. Eva was a girl who hung out with friends of his friends. They met at a party out late one night and they "hooked up" after hanging out together for a while when both of them were pretty drunk. After that, Eva started hanging out at Dirk's house, a college dump he rented with friends.

After a couple of months, Dirk and Eva saw each other almost every day. The two of them became friends and really liked each other a lot. Actually, Eva fell in love in with Dirk, but Dirk was mostly having a good time and didn't even stop to think about how he really felt about Eva. Eva was nice enough, but they never really talked about being "boyfriend and girlfriend" or being in an exclusive relationship. Dirk and Eva used the "withdrawal" method or "pull-out" method of birth control. "Pull-out" means Dirk was to not ejaculate semen inside of Eva's vagina during sex, so she wouldn't get pregnant. This was not very effective for many reasons, including: the guy not having very good ejaculatory control, or pre-ejaculation can impregnate a girl, or the guy just "goes for it" and doesn't pull out.

After three months of being together, Eva missed her period. Eva took a couple of home pregnancy tests, which were positive. Then she went to tell Dirk in person that she was pregnant. Eva was crying and completely hysterical. She was emotional, tearful, and looking to Dirk for some support.

Dirk was shocked. At first, he just tried to calm Eva down and talk to her, and he even held her while she cried. At first, Dirk tried to be nice. Then, it hit him. He started getting really scared about her being pregnant and frightened with the thought of his being a father.

How Do I Know When I'm Ready for Sex?

Dirk still had 2½ years of college left to complete before he could graduate and get a job. It suddenly hit him that he might have to quit college and get a job and start supporting the baby. Dirk didn't want to be a father, yet. He saw himself having children much, much later in his life, when he was making good money and he could have a house, a nice car, and he could take his kids to amusement parks and on vacations. Dirk was not, absolutely not, ready to be a father.

Dirk immediately knew he wanted Eva to have an abortion. Even though it was against his own religion teachings, Dirk still knew he wanted Eva to have an abortion. Dirk did not want Eva to be pregnant. He felt extremely strongly that he just wanted the whole problem to go away and not have to deal with the problem of a pregnancy, being a father, supporting a child, telling his parents, who were also Catholic and against abortion, or even the distant thought of getting married to Eva. Dirk liked Eva a lot, but he'd only known her for a few months. He thought a lot about Eva when he was away from her, but he didn't really know if he loved her, and he wasn't ready for marriage, which is what he thought his parents would expect him to do if he got a girl pregnant. Right away, he told Eva he wanted her to have an abortion.

Then, the problems started.

Eva, it turns out, while she was "pro-choice," which meant she agreed women should have the right to decide if they want to have an abortion, legally, she did not believe in abortion for herself. In fact, Eva was very much against having an abortion. Eva told Dirk that she would do almost anything for him, because she loved him, but she couldn't and wouldn't have an abortion.

Dirk was very surprised, to say the least. Dirk and Eva had never talked about what they would do if they had an unplanned pregnancy. Dirk had no idea how Eva felt toward abortion, or having children, or even adoption: he simply never thought about talking to her about what they would do if she became pregnant. Dirk became panicked, and he turned into a very ugly person toward Eva. He told her, of course, that he wanted her to have an abortion. He told her that he wasn't ready to be a father. He begged her to please consider that he couldn't help to support the child for at least 2 more years and he desperately wanted to finish college.

Eva, although she tried to be kind to him, was emotionally devastated. Since she was in love with Dirk, she had hoped that he also loved her and that somehow he would support her, at least emotionally, and do his best to help her take care of this child. Eva thought, since she and Dirk had practically been living together in his house for the past 2 months, that they would move in together and take care of the child together. Also, Eva told Dirk that she knew if she had an abortion, to her it would be killing a baby and she would be haunted by it for the rest of her life and she simply could not do it, ever.

Next, Dirk became angry. He began to emotionally manipulate and tried to coerce her into having an abortion. He was desperate and frightened and adamant that he didn't want any children at this time in his life, and he became very mean toward Eva. Dirk told Eva that he "would never have anything to do with her if she had this baby and didn't have an abortion." Dirk told her that he would never have anything to do with the child, that he would never support the child, that she was ruining his life, and pleaded with her repeatedly to have an abortion and to stop hurting him, if she had any shred of love for him in her body.

Eva told Dirk that she still loved him, but she had a baby inside her and she simply could not do this to a child. In reality, Eva was torn: she was only 18. She had no job, no education, no ability to support a child, and the father of the baby was completely rejecting and abandoning her. She even started thinking about having an abortion, even though every fiber in her body told her it was wrong. Simply, she didn't know how she would take care of a child, without the father helping her, and she never, never wanted to be a single mother. Dirk saw that Eva might be weakening and he told her he

How Do I Know When I'm Ready for Sex?

would pay for the abortion and "be there every step of the way." Dirk waited and prayed that Eva would agree to have an abortion.

But, Eva did not change her mind and she refused to agree to have an abortion. Soon, she turned to her family for support and told them about the pregnancy and how Dirk was treating her. Eva's parents were shocked and disappointed; however, they became surprisingly supportive of her and agreed to help her, no matter what. They, too, were not in favor of abortion, although they were not happy with her teenage pregnancy, either.

Finally, Eva told Dirk that if he wasn't going to have anything to do with her, unless she had an abortion, then he shouldn't call her anymore, because she was going to have the baby. Dirk and Eva went back and forth with talking and not speaking to each other during the pregnancy. After the time passed, when Eva couldn't have an abortion legally anymore, Dirk stopped, of course, emotionally manipulating her about abortion, but he was still very angry that he was going to become a father "against his will."

Eva gave birth to a healthy baby boy. Eva lived with her parents, who help to care for the child to this day, while she finishes her education. Dirk is still in college, and he works 20 hours a week, but he had to move home with his parents so he could pay his child support, in addition to taking student loans to pay for school. Dirk eventually got over his anger toward Eva for not having an abortion and "ruining his life." After the baby was born, he began to see his son and accepted parenthood. With the help of his parents, he continued college and helps Eva raise their child.

Option #1: Get an Abortion

An abortion is a legal medical procedure, early in a pregnancy, to remove a fetus, or a growing "baby," from a woman's uterus before it has grown enough to live on its own outside the womb. Many girls have conflicting feelings about abortion. A lot of guys will pressure girls into having an abortion, as in the last story of "Dirk." As you can see, regardless of your feelings, thoughts, and plans, the option of abortion is up to the girl.

The truth is that the vast majority of guys, teenage guys who are facing unplanned fatherhood, choose abortion as the #1 option to dealing with pregnancy. For teenage guys, 9 out of 10 of you will not be around by the end of the pregnancy when your child is born. The fact is that most teenage guys do not want to have children. They want their girlfriends or friends with benefits girl to have an abortion, and if she does have the baby, most teenage guys abandon teenage mothers and their children. Guys, this does not make you look very good here. This is one of the reasons guys get a bad reputation for the way they treat girls! Abandoning a pregnant girl hurts the girl, it hurts an innocent child who needs a dad, and really, it will hurt you, too.

It can and does hurt guys emotionally, too. Truthfully, some guys wish and pray that the girl will have an abortion and then are relieved when she does and its over, but more and more young women are choosing to keep their children, not opt for abortion, and will have your child. For some guys, it hurts them when they ask a girl to have an abortion, because it might be against their religion, or it might make them feel a sense of loss later in their life, especially if they have no other children, but even when they do later have a family.

You need to take some time here to reflect on your values about abortion. You must make sure that having an abortion is the right decision for you. Also, I strongly advise that you consider your girlfriend's values, as well, and how to support her. In Dirk's case, above, he felt guilty for putting so much pressure on Eva and hurting her over and over again by threatening her and abandoning her, when she was so scared and going through a pregnancy all alone.

For some girls and guys, there are spiritual considerations as well as emotional considerations in having an abortion. Some people feel that having an abortion is the same as murder—that is, that an abor-

115

tion is killing a baby. For some people, having an abortion is like getting rid of "extra cells" that do not need to grow in their body, that do not need to grow into a baby. In such a case, abortion may be the right decision for many teenage couples, and although there might be feelings of loss, there may be a relief when it appears to be the best choice for everyone. Some people say they feel a sense of loss throughout their life, but when you have a baby, you also have to take care of that child every day of it's life. You need to know your view on abortion and/or think it over and/or talk it over with someone. For some people, even more strongly for women, there are feelings of guilt and loss that last for years after having an abortion when it is the wrong decision for them, sometimes even if they think it is the right decision at the time of the procedure. If you do coerce a girl into having an abortion when she is strongly against it, that could be on your conscious for the rest of your life.

When you find out about a pregnancy, it is usually a big shock no matter what the circumstances. This means that you should really take some time to get your head back down to earth, so you can search your heart and mind and make the right decision for you. Sometimes talking to a minister, therapist, parent or friend may help you in weighing your options and feelings about abortion, and sometimes, the right decision at the time of the abortion is based on your gut feeling. However, as of right now, the decision for an abortion is the girls, not the guys, and there is nothing you can do about it.

Option #2: She Keeps the Baby

Once the decision is made that she will be continuing the pregnancy, you will need to start making the choice of whether or not you will be a part of your girlfriend's life, a part of the pregnancy, and/or a part of your child's life. As stated above, 9 out of 10 teenage guys are not be present by the end of the 9 month pregnancy, by the time their teenage girlfriend gives birth. Chances are very good that you will abandon your girlfriend and you will abandon your child and your child will not have a father.

Will this be you? Only you can make the choice.

Did you grow up with a Dad? How important was having a father in your life? What would you have done without him? If he wasn't there, how often did you long for a father to be there for you, on birthdays, holidays, or at your ball game? Did you ever make a vow that you would be a better dad?

One of the greatest gifts a Dad can give to his child is to love their mother. Mothers need caring, support, emotionally and financially, and help in raising children. Sometimes, they just need a listening ear. If you want to love your child, be loving to their mother, even if you are not in love with her. Even if you are not planning to be with the mother, she is the mother of your child and she deserves your respect and support, so she can be a good mom.

Whether you stay with the mom or not, you can choose to be a part of your child's life. As a teen dad, if you plan to be in this child's life, you will need to tell your family, and ask for their support. Your parents or guardians will need to be told, as they will eventually find out about it. For most teenagers, it is a very difficult thing to tell their mother and/or father or grandparents that their girlfriend is pregnant. Just imagine how difficult it might be to tell your parents that you are sexually active. Then imagine telling them that your girlfriend is pregnant—it's even harder. However, if you choose to be a part of your child's life, you will need the support of your family. If you family is no help, seek help through the church or even the local health department. Often, cities have programs to help teen dads be better fathers.

The (Ugly) Realities of Being a Teen Dad

1. You will have to pay child support. Even If you don't work, the court will assess an income for you based on minimum wage, and you'll have to pay something. Don't mess with child support: It will ruin the relationship with your child's mother; your child will know about it and won't respect you, and you will go to jail if you don't pay.

2. You will have visitation of your child on a court schedule, usually every other weekend.

3. You will not be able to party with your friends when you are caring for your child, because if you do care for your child, it is a 24-hour, 7-days-a-week, job.

4. If you are not married, the mother usually gets custody and is raising your child with her values and rules and you will be a visitor in your child's life.

5. You will have to deal with the mother of your child for the rest of your life. If you get along, great. If you don't, it is a constant source of irritation in your life for many years. This is the #1 reason fathers don't visit their children: they can't deal with the conflicts with the mother, not because they don't love their children.

6. Most teen fathers have female relatives who help them, like mothers and grandmothers, and they will want to control what you do with your child and life.

7. Your plans for your future of college, education, or training will be interrupted, will take much longer to accomplish, or will be difficult to accomplish due to time, even if you are highly motivated.

8. Future relationships may be affected by your having a child and having to pay your earnings to support your first child.

9. Your child can be given up for adoption, sometimes without your consent.

10. The chances of your child growing up in poverty are over 50%.

Option #3: Make Plans for Adoption

For many girls, after carrying a baby for nine months, emotionally it is very hard to give up a baby for adoption. The option of adoption, because you are unable to provide a child with the life you want to give him or her, is often a courageous act, and may be the best choice to meet the needs of your child. Unfortunately, some men and women suffer a sense of loss over their child for years, because of not knowing the whereabouts of their child or how the child is being cared for, wishing they could have raised their child, and just missing their child.

Open adoptions can help with these problems of loss, because you know who the child is with and you may obtain pictures and information about the child as he or she grows up. It can be very heartwarming to know your child is well taken care of and you have helped a couple fulfill their dreams of having a family. Many loving, eagerly awaiting adoptive parents are quite ready and eager to make a wonderful home for your child and can provide many opportunities in life you can not provide your child as a teenager.

Yet, in some cases, children who are adopted feel a sense of loss regarding their parents, and they feel rejected or abandoned by their biological parents. Although, in the balance of all thoughts and emotions, an adoption may be the best thing for a father, mother and child, there are frequently emotional consequences for the everyone, including your parents. On the other hand, there are emo-tional consequences of raising a child every day, when you are not prepared to take on the very huge responsibility.

Option #4: Get Married or Live Together

Teenage marriages have a lot of problems and suffer a high divorce rate. Thirty percent of teens who marry, where the bride is under 18, end in divorce within 5 years; however, that means that 70% survive! Taking care of yourself as a teenager can be very difficult for the most mature and skilled person. It is difficult to get adjusted to taking personal responsibility for all parts of your life on your own. Just think of some of the conflicts you have now with your parents: keeping your room clean, doing your homework, and hav-ing money for fun. If you get married, you are suddenly responsible for *all* of these things yourself. On top of this, you will be responsible for an infant's life, too. This is a lot of responsibility for the aver-age teenager. In addition, a lot of teenage relationships do not work out, often because the couple is too immature to deal with all of the problems of finances and taking care of a baby, not to mention know how to treat someone right, fight fairly, and work out problems with good communication. A lot of teenage couples don't stay together because at that age, people break up and want to date other people and cheat on each other.

The responsibility of supporting yourself at 18, even if you have financial support from your family or from state welfare, is often too much for a young adult or couple. The strain of having a baby crying for hours a day, getting sick, needing constant attention, with the responsibility of working and taking care of your own home or apart-ment, or worst yet, living with your parents, can break up the most determined and loving couple. If you decide to get married or to live together independently, be prepared to grow up fast, get support from your family and friends, and be ready to put the needs of your child first. With support from your family and community, some teen relationships and marriages can and do survive, and after the first few years, after you realize you have to grow up and mature, it can become much easier, especially if you love one another. My parents married when they were pregnant at 18 and 19 years old. They had three kids by the time my dad graduated from college three years later, and ten children altogether. This year, they are celebrating their 50th anniversary. It can work, it can be amazingly wonderful, it can be very hard at times, but true love can survive! Miracles happen.

7. AM I READY TO USE BIRTH CONTROL AND PRACTICE SAFER SEX?

If you want to be ready to have sex, you must be ready to use birth control and practice safer sex *each and every time you have sex*, unless you want to risk being a teenage father and risk your physical health. As you can see, from the stories above, you do NOT want to risk pregnancy! Even though NO birth control is 100% effective, Chapter Seven discusses different types of birth control, as well as ways to be sexually active, without having sexual intercourse.

One of the biggest mistakes that guys make, when it comes to sex. is either choosing not to use birth control or leaving the birth control up to the girl.

Rusty's Story—Part 2

> Remember Rusty, who we met in Chapter One, whose goal on his 15th birthday was to get laid? Well, he finally got over his awkward, embarrassing, desperate stage of seeking any kind of sex with any kind of girl, and finally got his first girlfriend when he was 16. Rusty was a virgin and she was a virgin, so Rusty didn't think they had to worry about using condoms. Rusty figured as long as neither of them

had had sex with anyone else, they were safe from STDs. For birth control, she told him she was on the pill, so he didn't worry about it. Rusty stayed with his first girlfriend for almost a year, and they didn't have any problems: no pregnancies, no STDs. In the end, she broke it off with Rusty and he was pretty tore up about it, and he decided to go wild with sex after that.

After his break up, Rusty became a bit of a dog and started to try to have sex with any girl who would have sex with him. Now, Rusty had a problem: He was used to not using condoms for a whole year and he decided he liked not using condoms and he wasn't going to wear one! Even if the girl asked him to wear one, he refused and said he didn't have anything (which he didn't) and he'd convince the girl to have sex without a condom. Also, when it came to birth control, Rusty left the birth control up to the girl: He was used to his girlfriend being on the pill and "taking care of things." Also, in the back of his mind, he figured it was the girl's problem if she got pregnant, if she didn't take the pill, and she could get an abortion, if there was a problem. Rusty's best friend's girlfriend had an abortion when she got pregnant, so Rusty just figured if some girl got pregnant, she'd have an abortion, too. Over the next year, Rusty had sex with a reported 6 different girls (he might have been exaggerating, though). Rusty bragged to everyone that he "never wore a condom" and he "never would!"

The trouble started with an STD. Rusty broke out in blisters all over his groin area, including on his testicles and on the bottom of his penis. He had about 20 itching, painful blisters, he broke out into a fever and his groin ached so bad, he finally went to the doctor. Within minutes, the doctor told Rusty he had gotten herpes.

After he got some treatment for the herpes, Rusty was told he had to call every girl he had sex with and tell them that they might have been exposed to the STD.

For Rusty, every phone call was a wake-up call. Every girl was so mad at him that by the time he finished calling the third person,

Rusty thinks everyone in town knew he had herpes (you know how girls can blow up a phone line). By the time he called the fourth girl, she already knew and she starting screaming at him on the phone, too. The next two weeks were the worst two weeks of his life: Not only was he in pain and uncomfortable with his blisters (for about 10 days, despite the medication), but it was like he had leprosy. No girls wanted to talk to him and no girls were going to go out with him for a long time.

Fortunately, Rusty did get lucky, that none of the girls had gotten pregnant. However, after everyone found out about the herpes, he never "got laid" again for the rest of high school. Eventually, Rusty decided to move out of town after he finished high school. He also decided to change his mind and use condoms in the future. He isn't sure how many girls he gave herpes to (he thinks maybe one, but he thinks she might have been lying) and he felt really bad about it. Rusty was also mad that he got it, because with herpes you can treat the symptoms, but you have it for life (see more about herpes in Chapter Seven). Rusty also has to tell every future sexual partner that he has herpes. He's very ashamed of having it and he's afraid he'll never find someone to have sex with him again.

Rusty was now up to making at least 5 of the common sexual mistakes. He went out with anyone who would go out with him, he didn't practice safe sex, he didn't practice birth control, he didn't think about the girl's feelings, and he probably cheated on at least one girl if he had sex with six different girls in a year. Rusty has to live with at least one of his mistakes for the rest of his life.

Before having any sexual contact, you need to know how sexual behavior can be risky to your health, and how to protect yourself from these risks as much as possible. Chapter Seven discusses sexually transmitted diseases (STDs) and birth control more fully. While many schools provide some information on STDs and risky sexual behavior, it is important to know how to distinguish unsafe, safer,

How Do I Know When I'm Ready for Sex?

and safe sex. Some STDs can kill you, others stay with you for life, and others are painful but will go away with medical attention. You should also be aware that there is really no such thing as absolutely safe sex. Abstinence is the only sure way not to risk getting an STD or pregnancy. However, you can learn about how to have safer sex.

If you are lucky, you will have or have had a good sex ed class in school. Yet, even the best sex ed courses in high school will not tell you everything about STDs, often because they are restricted by laws to talk about everything you need to know. For example, you can get an STD without having sexual intercourse, such as gonorrhea of the throat from giving oral sex. You can also get genital herpes by receiving oral sex from someone who has a fever blister on or in their mouth. In short, you need to educate yourself thoroughly about birth control and STDs prior to having any sexual contact with another person.

Do I Know How to Get and Use Condoms to Protect Myself Against STDs?

Condoms can be used to prevent STDs. They do not protect you from every kind of sexually transmitted disease, but they have been proven to help reduce the risk significantly. Condoms can be purchased at drug stores and some grocery stores. You do not have to be 18 to buy condoms. There are many different types and brands of condoms. All it takes is money and a way to get to a store to buy them, or *you can go to your local health clinic department or teen clinic to get free ones.* Some people are very shy about buying condoms, but you must be able to be confident enough to buy condoms to be ready to have sex.

Am I Prepared to Use Birth Control Every Time I Have Sex?

- Do you or your girlfriend know how to get birth control?
- Do we really know what kinds of birth control are available?
- Are you responsible enough to use it every time you have sex?

- Are you responsible in other ways in your life, like with school-work or doing what you're supposed to do every day, which would indicate that you are mature enough to take birth control seriously as an every day responsibility?
- Are you willing to take responsibility for birth control yourself and not just count on your girlfriend to take care of it?
- Are you prepared to talk to your parents about getting birth control if you can't take care of your birth control needs for yourself?
- Do you realize that all types of birth control have a failure rate?
- Do you know which type of birth control is the best one for you?

A big mistake that guys make is counting on their girlfriend to take care of the birth control. For one, girls can lie. A girl might want to get pregnant and you will be trapped into being a father (or paying for an abortion)! Or she may too embarrassed to talk to you truthfully about birth control, too embarrassed or unable to go to a doctor, or she may not be able to get or take birth control. Many girls can not tell their parents they are sexually active, or they could get grounded for life and then they would never see you again! The only way you can control whether or not a girl gets pregnant is if YOU control the birth control. A condom or abstinence or "withdrawal" methods are the only way that a guy can control birth control. A girl can say she's on the pill, when she's not. Or, she can be irresponsible in taking it correctly. Using "pull-out" or withdrawal is not effective: 30% of the time, the girl will get pregnant within a year! Using a condom is the best way to avoid STDs and control birth control, if you choose to be sexually active. Are you prepared to get them and use them every time? More information is given in Chapter Seven, on birth control and unplanned pregnancy.

8. AM I COMFORTABLE ENOUGH WITH MY GIRLFRIEND TO TALK ABOUT SEX?

Often, many teenage couples are too shy to really talk about sex. Or, they simply don't take the time to develop a relationship that involves sexual communication, before becoming sexually active. However, it is important to have open communication with your partner in order to be ready for sex and avoid negative sexual consequences, such as pregnancy, STDs, or even misunderstandings about having mutual sexual consent, that is, making sure she said yes and means it. As a guy, you certainly don't want to get into trouble by getting accused of sexually molesting or raping someone because you didn't have a clear sexual communication and understanding. In order to be ready for sex, you need to know that you can talk about sex comfortably with each other.

Besides talking about sex, there are many things you should be able to talk to your girlfriend about before you have a sexual relationship.

Can We Talk?

1. First, ask yourself if you can talk about other things besides sex.
2. Second, do you feel comfortable and accepted enough by your girlfriend to believe that she will take your opinions and feelings seriously?
3. Third, do you trust her enough to talk about your every day life as well as your biggest secrets and fears?

> If you can't feel comfortable talking about life in general, you are not ready to talk about sex, and you're not ready for sex.

A lot of guys don't really know what to say to a girl, or where to start, nevertheless talk about sex. Look at the topics below. Start by talking about general things, like school and work, then move on to more personal topics, like friends and family or your dreams and goals, and then how you feel toward one another, and perhaps, on to your thoughts and feelings about sex.

We're Just Talking

- Do you talk about school?

- Do you talk about your jobs?

- Does she know about your family? Does she understand and/or accept your family situation?

- Does she accept and know your friends?

- Have you talked about your dreams and goals in life?

- Have you talked about your likes and dislikes regarding interests and activities?

- Have you talked about your likes and dislikes about clothing and dress?

- Have you talked about your likes and dislikes about food and going out to eat?

- Have you talked about your likes and dislikes about movies, TV, or books?

- Would you call her when you have a crisis, like if your car breaks down?

- Do you feel like you can talk to her about almost anything, including your values about sex?

- Can you talk to her about how you feel, such as liking her?

- Can you tell her if you like something sexually or not? Can she tell you?

- Can you talk about being a virgin or previous sexual partners, because of the risk of STDs.

- Can you tell her you want to wear a condom?

- You should be able to talk about birth control, make decisions about what to use, and decide together to use it.

- You need to talk about the potential consequences of pregnancy.

- Can you agree with each other about having other sexual partners or being "exclusive," meaning you don't date other people or have sex with anyone?

- Can you feel comfortable saying no? Can she feel comfortable saying no to you?

128

A girl can't say yes to sex until she can really say no.

Think long and hard about this statement. If she can't say no to sex, then she really isn't comfortable and confident enough to say yes and mean it! Although sexual communication may be embarrassing at first, if you do not have it, there will be a lot more problems later. If you can't talk to your girlfriend openly about sex, you are really not ready to have sex!

9. CAN MY GIRLFRIEND AND I LEGALLY HAVE SEX?

You need to be concerned with whether or not you and your girlfriend can legally have sex, based on your ages. There are usually two laws that are important when it comes to sex, based on your ages.

- It is against the law for an adult to have sex with a minor.
- It is against the law to have sex with anyone who is not yet the "age of consent."

In almost all states, it's against the law and called "statutory rape" if an adult has sex with a minor. That is, a person over the age of 18, considered an adult, has sex with a person under 18, considered a minor. Statutory rape means either the person having sex has not reached the legal "age of consent" in your state, or is an adult having sex with a minor. For example, in South Carolina and Michigan, the age of consent is 16. This means that it is against the law to have sex with someone who has not yet reached the age of 16. Even if two people love each other, and even if they both say they consented to a sexual relationship, a guy or a girl can get in very serious legal trouble for statutory rape, including being arrested for sexual assault and being labeled a sex offender for life. Most 18-year-old guys know what the term "jailbait" stands for, and you should, too: it means a young girl may be terrifically tempting, but she is too young to have sex with, and he can go to jail if he does.

The Legal Bottom Line

1. You both need to be the "age of consent" to legally have a sexual relationship. This age varies from state to state, but 16 is the average age. Call your local sheriff's office and ask about the age of sexual consent in your state or country.
2. You both must be minors who are the legal age of consent or you must both be adults.
3. If one of you is a minor and the other is an adult, then it is not legal to have a sexual relationship, and the adult can get into legal trouble, even if you love each other and the minor "consented" to the sexual relationship. If you really love each other, you will both accept the legal reality of this situation, and

act responsibly with each other. For example, if a minor gets pregnant, and the father is an adult, he can face legal charges of statutory rape for his actions.

The most common situation where someone is charged with statutory rape is when an adult male has sex with a minor female, who is not of the age of consent. For example, when a 25-year-old man has sex with a 13-year-old girl, the man is going to serve time in jail for statutory rape. However, an adult woman who has sex with a boy can also be charged with statutory rape, like the recent media cases of male students having sex with their teachers. The most publicized case is against Mary Kay Leturneau, who was in her mid-thirties and had sex with her 12-year-old, 6th grade student. The teacher got pregnant and went to jail. Even though they both said they were in love, when she got out of jail, they got back together and she got pregnant a second time with his child. She went back to jail for 7 years.

A young man needs to beware of being with an "underage" girl, especially in interracial relationships, and especially when the girl gets pregnant. It is not uncommon for a black male over the age of 18 to be charged with statutory rape when a white girl has gotten pregnant and her parents got angry and went to the police. In such a case, the young man will be labeled a sex offender for life, even though he might have been 18 and she was 15 and they professed their love for each other. If only one of you is an adult, someone can get in trouble—serious trouble.

In some states, once a girl or guy has reached the "age of consent," generally being around 16, the law of "sex with a minor" is often not enforced. For example, in South Carolina, once a girl is 16, or the age of consent, that even if the guy is not a minor, if he is a teenager of 17, 18, or 19, the police often do not enforce the law of "sex with a minor." If there is a really big age difference, like a 35-year-old having sex with a 16-year-old, then the police might try to enforce the law of sex with a minor, but generally, once a person has reached the "age of consent," and both parties are teenagers, the "sex with a minor" law is seldom enforced.

Also, if both teenagers are below the "age of consent," meaning two teens are under the age of 16 (or age of consent in your state), *neither or both* can be charged with statutory rape. In all the cases I have seen, when both were under the age of consent, no charges were filed, since either person could be charged with statutory rape and parents don't want *their* child to get into legal trouble.

> Legal troubles start when one person is a minor or under the age of consent and the other person is an adult.

Legal matters aside, age and maturity level can strongly affect your relationship. Most teenagers find that they get along better in a relationship, and especially a sexual relationship, if they are closer in age and maturity level. How close you need to be in age can vary, but generally, two years is a good guideline and three years is pushing it.

Maturity levels vary a lot among people, regardless of their age. In general, girls tend to be about two years ahead of guys emotionally. As a result, many girls want to date older guys, because emotionally they may relate to each other better. For a 15-year-old girl and 15-year-old guy, some interests may be the same, but you may be very far apart in having an emotional connection. For example, a 15-year-old girl may be want to have deep, intimate conversations about feelings, while as a 15-year-old guy, you may still be more interested in playing video games. Having similar maturity levels usually means that you will have more interests in common and you may be more compatible emotionally than not. So, it's not uncommon for younger girls to want to date older guys. If you're the older guy and you have a sexual relationship with a girl who is not of the age of consent, you risk serious trouble. Also, as an older guy, you might be ready for a sexual relationship, but she's not. Pressuring a girl into having sex, even if she is "the age of consent," can still be legally viewed as rape, when she's a minor. Hopefully, with maturity, you can decide together if you are both ready for sex and consider if you can have a sexual relationship without someone getting into trouble legally.

10. WOULD I HAVE SEX IF I WEREN'T DRUNK OR HIGH?

Different than the rest of the questions in this quiz, often this question presents itself suddenly, in a moment when you are in a situation that you are drinking or using drugs. You can make a decision *now*, to *not* make a decision about sex unless you are sober, and this may help prevent many problems. One of the biggest mistakes that teens make, when it comes to sex, is deciding that they are ready for sex when they are drunk or high. It is just simply easier to forget your "conditions" for sex, or to minimize their importance, when you are intoxicated. Most of my clients, both teens and adults, have made at least one sexual mistake, at some point in their lives, because they had too much to drink or, as the song says, "because I got high."

You are much less likely to make good decisions about sex when you are drunk or high. Also, drugs and alcohol can affect your feelings of attraction and intensify your sexual excitement, or bluntly put, can make you feel horny when you normally wouldn't feel that way. Let's say one of your conditions for having a sexual relationship is that you will *always* use a condom until you are engaged or married. When you're drunk, you might decide this condition for sex isn't nearly as important as wanting to be with some really hot girl. Or you may be too high to bother taking the time to go to the place you keep a condom, or remember where it is, or to get it in the heat of the moment. One of your conditions for sex might be that you have to have a strong attraction to someone before you make out with them. You might find yourself attracted to someone you would never have been attracted to when you were sober, leaving you feeling very embarrassed the next day when everyone finds out who you hooked up with.

Coyote Ugly

Ever hear the term, "coyote ugly?" It's a "humorous" term for the mistake of drunken sexual stupidity. Coyote ugly refers the appearance of a girl you had sex with when you were both very drunk and slept together. The next morning you wake up and realize your sexual partner was so ugly, which you didn't notice the night before when you were totally wasted, that now, in the morning, you are so embarrassed that you desperately want to get out of the bedroom. Unfortunately, you're still in bed, and she's laying on your arm, but if you move it she'll wake up and remember you had sex with her. So, instead, you'd rather chew your arm off, like a coyote, to escape the scene unnoticed.

133

Very often, when people choose to have virgin sex when they are drunk or high, they regret their choices the next day, when they're sober. You might consent to having sexual experiences or sex for the first time when you are drunk or high, but if you were sober, you would have *never* had a sexual encounter with that person, or in that place, or at that time. You might just let things happen and not use your usual good judgment or physical ability to say no. Sometimes, you are just too drunk to care about yourself. Sometimes, people get date raped because they have less ability to avoid a situation or to stop it from happening. Date rape will be discussed further in Chapter Nine. Sometimes, people are so intoxicated that they black out and do not remember anything of the sexual encounter.

Did you know? If you have sex with a girl who was too drunk to legally consent to sex, you can be charged with date rape in some states!

If you choose to drink or use drugs, you need to be very careful about the situations in which you put yourself. Parties are terribly dangerous settings for regrettable sexual situations. Better yet, stay away from drugs and alcohol in dating situations, especially until you have more experience with both sex and using alcohol. As a teenager, you probably don't know your drinking limits, and it is not a good idea to get into dating situations while you are also experimenting with alcohol.

Calhoun's Story

Calhoun was planning on waiting until he got married to have sex. He made a vow of abstinence until marriage. It was his values that he saved his virginity for the girl he would spend the rest of his life. At his very first frat party his freshman year in college, he got totally drunk, and remembers only sketches of the night. The next morning, he was in bed with a girl his frat brothers set him up with, knowing he was a virgin, because they thought it would be funny "to get him laid." Calhoun had only met the girl once and realized they had sex when he woke up next to her, the next day. He felt very ashamed of losing his virginity this way, and he was very angry with his friends. For a long time, he brushed it off and got over being angry at his friends for his fraternity "hazing," until he met a girl and fell in love, a year later. He felt very embarrassed and sad to tell her he wasn't a virgin, and he regretted not "saving himself," for her.

Make virgin sex sober sex.

FIVE

THE BEGINNING OF SEX

Sex begins before you are born. William Masters was the "father of sex therapy," and he became interested in sex as a field of study when he was a medical intern delivering babies in the 1950s. Dr. Masters was surprised to see that some male babies were born with erect penises. He was quite surprised and asked the doctor in charge if that had ever happened before. The doctor told him no, that it was just an unusual thing. But Dr. Masters found out, after attending many births, that it was a *common* happening! This motivated Dr. Masters to become interested in the study of sex. Later, he found out that baby boys get erections even before they are born, when they are developing in their mother's wombs. This means that babies are sexual beings from before birth! Later, Dr. Masters found out that girls were wired sexually at least from birth because infant girls have lubrication or wetness in their vaginas! However, most parents do not think about their children as sexual beings even when the children reach their teens. So many times, adults expect that their kids should "save sex for marriage" and not have sexual feelings, thoughts, or behaviors until they are adults or married, but people have sexual feelings from the very beginning of their lives.

You are wired for sex from birth, and it's normal.

FIRST SEXUAL FEELINGS

People are often curious about when children begin to have sexual feelings. A common question is, "When do people begin to masturbate?" The answer is: "When their diaper comes off." Often, this is in the bathtub prior to a baby's potty training. Babies stretch their arms out all around them: in the air, on the bath toy, in their eyes, on their toes, and at some point, they touch their genitals. They realize this feels *good*. So they touch themselves again and again. Some parents react by moving their baby's hands off their genitals because they perceive self-touch to be "*bad*" or "*dirty*." But why is self-touching bad? Many parents simply do not think that a child should have sexual awareness of even a rudimentary sort, like touching him or herself. This is where the "Sex is *bad*" message starts. Parents move their baby's hands away because their hand is in the "wrong place." The result is that this place, the child's own genital area, is perceived as wrong from infancy, in spite of the fact that sexual feelings are natural and begin even before birth. Yet, for some people and religious teachings, genital touch, let alone actual sexual behavior, is suddenly supposed to be right only after the rite of marriage, right?

When boys are 2 and 3 years old, it is common for them to run around the house naked and laughing, using their penis as a guide, pointing it in every direction they want to go. Sometimes they yell out, "I have a PENIS!" Most parents laugh, and eventually teach their children to be private, wear clothes, and to only touch their "privates" in their room or bathroom, when they're alone. Yet, for some parents, it is upsetting to have a child openly touch themselves or even to be naked. Sadly, some children are harshly scolded to "stop touching yourself down there" or "that's dirty."

This is the beginning of sex, when a child is told that sexual touch or pleasuring is bad or dirty or OK, which is the beginning of the association of shame or joy with sex. A big problem in our society is that many children are taught from the beginning of their lives that even nudity, let alone the natural sexual functioning of their bodies, is *wrong*. For a lot of you teenagers reading this book, you may have one or more memories of being told that nudity or touching yourself is wrong, which feels shameful. Sometimes there is no gentle guidance in teaching you about *privacy* and learning lessons on the wonders of sex.

Michael's Story

Michael had a very embarrassing incident when he was caught masturbating.

Michael first masturbated when he was 13, and got his own room. Michael was very happy to finally have privacy, since he'd always shared a room with his younger brother. Michael loved his new bedroom he moved into after his parents finally refinished the basement, including a private bathroom.

Michael found some old condoms in his parent's room, deep in the bowels of their bathroom cabinet, which was more of a time capsule than a closet. He found an old, huge box of pre-lubricated condoms that looked like they hadn't been used since before he was conceived. He took the whole box.

He began to masturbate, using the old, still quite lubricated condoms. His bed in the basement was right next to a small access door to the sump pump. The sump pump was an emergency water pump, which would drain the water in the basement, in case of heavy rains or floods. Michael was oblivious to the purpose and use of the sump pump, because it had never been used or rained or flooded in their basement. Using the easy access door right next to his bed, he would stash the used condoms through the little door, and into the well of the sump pump, thinking one day he'd clean them all out.

That spring, it rained and rained and rained. All over the city, people were reporting flooding in their homes or basements, to which Michael was, again, totally oblivious. That night, Michael's parents went downstairs to check on the basement, to see if it had flooded. Michael's mom got to the bottom of the stairs first and immediately saw that there was 6 inches of water on the brand new carpet, and all across the floor of the basement. The carpet was totally destroyed and it cost $1,500 to just have it put in. But then, she received a shock.

Floating on the top of the water, were little, round, bright whitish colored circles, with tails. They were all over the basement floor: little round plastic looking things, that stood out in contrast to the navy blue carpet. She walked a few feet onto the basement floor and saw more of them, floating out from Michael's room. She reached down and picked up one of the circular floaters, placing it in her hand.

Then, she let out a loud scream!

Michael's dad came running down the stairs, through the pool of freezing cold water and rushing to his wife's side.

"What is the matter?" he shouted, concerned.

"There are used condoms floating all over the basement floor, and they're coming from *your* son's room!"

All of Michael's used condoms, a few dozen of them, that he had stashed in the well of the sump pump, had blocked the drainage of water and the activation of the sump pump. As water had filled the well, instead of the pump turning on and draining water, the condoms acted like a stopper in a kitchen sink. The water filled the well and then flooded over into the basement, for hours of rain and rain and rain, and swamped the basement floor. Slowly, the condoms had floated upwards and rested on to the top of the water, drifting in the sea of water throughout the rooms.

When Michael came home from school that day, he entered the kitchen, where his parents sat at the kitchen table. They looked up to him and just stared in silence. They didn't look happy. His stomach suddenly sank a foot and he got a huge lump in his throat. He knew the looks, he just didn't know why.

Dad said, "The basement flooded today. You need to go downstairs and clean up the mess."

Michael answered, slightly scared and slightly belligerent, "Why do I have to clean it up? I didn't make the rain flood the basement!"

Dad answered flatly, devoid of emotion, which was really scary, "You'll see and we'll talk later."

Ohmigod! Micheal did not like, never did, and dreaded the "We'll talk later," speech.

He was happy to be dismissed from THAT conversation and he turned on his heels and ran downstairs to his room, his sanctuary, and hoped his stuff wasn't ruined from the flood. He didn't get to the bottom stair, before he saw three round vivid objects, looking like small dead fish floating in the water, glowing under the bright white lightbulbs.

He died. He died right then and there. He sunk into a fetal position right there on the stairway, hugging his knees to his chest and falling sideways until his limp head hit the wall. He couldn't breathe. He just stared ahead of him to the bottom of the stairs, watching his fate drift in front of him.

Michael's father opened the door to the basement, standing above him, like a shadowy Freddy Krueger figure, with the light behind him, looking down at his next, cornered victim. Time stopped. Nobody spoke or breathed. It was like a time warp that Michael didn't want to get out of.

His dad broke the silence and began to descend down the stairs, closing in on him, quietly, like a panther toward prey. Michael was sure he would die of embarrassment, if his Dad didn't kill him first.

Dad sat down next to Michael and put his arm around him, and gave him two pats, exactly two. That was the two pat finish that he had felt before from his Dad that said, "It's OK."

All Dad said was, "It's OK, son, just clean it up, and use toilet paper and a garbage can next time." And then, they laughed.

MASTURBATION

You can always have sex with someone you love: yourself!

Masturbation is having sex with yourself, or touching yourself in a sexual way alone or with a intimate partner present. How you touch yourself in a sexual way is completely up to you and what you want to try and/or explore. Research shows that 75% of guys have masturbated by the age of 15 (and half of girls). Although most teenage guys do masturbate, not all do.

One of the biggest thing that happens for guys is when they cross the line from touching or pleasuring themselves, as most people do, to ejaculating, or becoming "comers." When guys reach the age of 12 or 13, they will experiencing ejaculation, which means they ejaculate semen or "come" after sexual stimulation, from rubbing or pulling or humping or touching their penis. Sometimes ejaculation happens for the first time in a nocturnal emission, or ejaculating in your sleep (see below for "wet dreams"). Some guys find this experience shocking or scary, as well as pleasurable and exciting. You do not need to be worried or concerned, but know that you have changed into being more of a man. And, at this time, many guys begin to experiment with masturbation more often.

Some families disagree with masturbation, for personal or usually religious reasons. Some religions believe masturbation is a sin. Some of the religious doctrine that believe masturbation is sinful goes back to the out-dated scientific writings (think: Old Testament times) that reported that each drop of semen contained miniature people

140

in them, and a man planted the "seed" or semen into the woman during sex to cause pregnancy. Hence, if you "spilled the seed," you were committing murder. Since murder is breaking was one of the ten commandments, masturbation was a sin. Modern science has disproved this belief, recognizing that semen is like a seed, because it must join with an egg to make a baby. Regardless of religious belief, most guys still masturbate, but some feel guilty about it. Prior to the 1960's, most medical writings supported myths of masturbation, some of which are still believed today, none of which are true.

Masturbation Myths

- It will make you go blind
- You will go straight to hell when you die
- Girls know when you've done it
- It will lead to insanity
- You will have underdeveloped sex organs (small balls)
- Parents know when you've done it

Since 75 to 95% of the population did not go blind or insane, sex researchers started studying masturbation. They found no research to show that masturbation is harmful to you mentally or sexually, unless you develop a sexual addiction. A sex addiction which means you can't stop when you want to or you are harming yourself. Some people say, "See, you can get a sexual addiction, so that is why it is wrong and harmful to masturbate." That is like saying, "See you can get a food addiction, so don't eat." We all know we have to eat, and we all know now that sexual feelings are normal human drives, like hunger. Typically, sex and eating are normal parts of living, although you don't have to have sex to live (you might just feel that way sometimes!).

Some guys are worried that they might masturbate too much. So, how much is "too much?" One young guy asked his dad, "What would happen if I masturbated 10 times a day?" His father answered, "Why would you *want* to?" To some young guys, masturbating is like getting a new toy: it is awful fun to play with for a while. Some guys "test" their virility and make a personal contest out of it, trying to find out how many times they can ejaculate or come in one day. Temporary fixations on masturbation are pretty common and it isn't going to hurt you. Eventually, you're likely to get tired of it, and like the dad, wonder why any one would want to spend that much time with masturbation. Yet, masturbation isn't just for adolescence. Most men masturbate all throughout their lives: sometimes when they are in relationships, sometimes when they are married, and sometimes not.

PORNOGRAPHY

When the subject of masturbation comes up, the subject of pornography follows. With the Internet, despite parental controls, most guys can access and have looked at pornography. A lot of mothers, as well as fathers, feel pornography is wrong or sinful. Some people, especially women, feel pornography is an exploitation of the women who are photographed. Pornography is seen as demeaning toward women because it portrays women as sexual objects, instead of people with feelings. Many people feel pornography is a vulgar portrayal of sexuality, rather than sexuality being a physical, emotional, and physical expression of love between two people, so they believe that pornography is inappropriate for teenagers (or anyone).

Vance's Story

Vance was the youngest of 6 children, including 3 older brothers. Before the time of the Internet, most young guys got their naked pictures or pornography from magazines. When Vance's next to oldest brother, Tim, was about to move out to go to college, Vance was very sad. He was very close to Tim and Vance would be left at home with only his two older sisters. At 14, Vance was really down that Tim was leaving. For the weeks before he left home, Tim told Vance, "Hey, don't worry about my leaving. When I go, I'm leaving you a big secret present." Vance was very curious about this mysterious present, but Tim wouldn't let on or tell him anything about it. Whenever Vance would start getting bummed out about Tim leaving or talking about going off to college, Tim would look at him, and wink at him or smile or nod his head or tell him directly, "Don't worry about me leaving, I'm leaving something behind, just between you and me, that will remind you of me and you'll be very happy about it." It was Tim's way of cheering Vance up and telling him not to be upset over his leaving, even though Vance was trying to hide his feelings.

Vance started to get over thinking about Tim leaving and starting wondering, with desperate curiosity what his brother could be leaving him. Although Vance was excited that he was going to get his own room soon, for the first time in his life, he knew *that* wasn't the surprise, he'd known that for years! The few days before Tim left, he almost started teasing Vance about the secret surprise. Tim would raise his eyebrows and taunt Vance, like it was a secret game, but he wouldn't let on, even a tiny little bit, about what the surprise might be.

The morning of the day Tim was leaving for college, he woke up very early, tore the covers off of Vance's bed, and jumped on him, probably for the last time before he left home for good, and punched him, kind of hard and kind of playfully in the stomach to wake his little brother up. Vance shook his head, tried to hide under his pillow, and go back to sleep. One more punch and Vance finally jumped out of bed, about ready to kill his brother. Then, Tim ran off and began to lead Vance to the basement, watching behind and around both of them, to make sure no one was looking. In their basement, it had the old time finished wood paneled walls and "drop ceilings," which were ceiling tiles set in rectangle metal frames, to make a basement ceiling. Tim lead Vance into the middle of the basement, and crawled up on top of the pool table, standing right up on the middle of the table. Tim reached up to the ceiling, and lifted up one of the ceiling tiles, reaching his hand along the topside of the roof of the basement.

Then, Tim pulled out a magazine. It was a Penthouse magazine. And he threw it at Vance. Vance's eyes opened wide. He quickly looked around again to make sure no one was looking, then he grabbed the magazine, opened it to the centerfold, spread it all the way out. His eyes lit up, but all he could say was, "Wow!"

Tim smiled. Then he told Vance to get up on the pool table and look for himself. There was a huge stack of a magazine collection, with at least 50 magazines, hidden in the ceiling of the basement. Vance started nodding his head up and down and up and down and all he could say was, "Oh, yeah!"

Tim explained to Vance that he got the collection from his next to older brother, when he left for college, who got the collection from their oldest brother, when he left for the Army, 10 years earlier. Tim smiled and told Vance to take good care of it. When Tim left that afternoon, Vance had a big smile on his face. No tears, just big hugs good-bye.

A year and a half later, Tim and Vance's parents had a Christmas party. It was held in their basement, and all the neighbors were invited. Many couples from their middle class neighborhood, where his parents had lived for 18 years and raised 6 kids, were sharing holiday cheer. That is, until the men got a bit excited and animated playing a game of pool, in the middle of the basement. One of the guys missed a shot and threw his head back and swung his arms and pool stick up high in the air in a funny gesture of frustration. Then it happened. The pool stick hit one of the lightweight, foam ceiling tiles, lifting it up in the air.

Much to everyone's surprise, the center of the room began to rain magazines. Tens and tens of magazines, with pictures of naked women, and breasts and buttocks and legs and more breasts, came flying down around the pool table. Everything seemed to happen as if it were in slow motion, because suddenly the air of the room was swallowed into the heavy gasps of the women—and men—while the pictures landed softly on top of the pool table and the floor. Right there, in the middle of their 1978 Christmas party, celebrating the birth of their Lord, Jesus Christ, were 50 or so Playboys, Penthouse, and Hustler magazines. Vance's mother looked over to her husband, and (while still seemingly in silent, slow motion) he was violently shaking his head back and forth, voicing over the muffled screams, "They're not MINE!"

After a moment of silence, all that could be heard was one loud scream in his mother's voice. "VAAAANNNNCCCCCCE!!!!!!"

The taboo and shock of pornography has not lessened in the past 30 years: just the delivery has changed, from magazines to websites. Nevertheless, most parents remain as opposed to porn as they were years ago. Even today, although Vance's parents have long since moved away, the legacy of Vance's family's 1978 Christmas party lives as a legend among the six childrens' childhood stories as one of the horrors and neighborhood humiliations that "the boys," caused the family. Today, they laugh about it—at least the boys do. I don't know about the girls.

As a sex therapist, one of my biggest concerns with pornography is that guys get most of their first sex education from the adult film industry. Real life sexuality is very, very different from pornography. Unrealistic expectations about women's bodies, what type of things women want to do, and the relationship that leads to sex (vs. casual porn sex) in real life can give guys the wrong idea about sharing love and sex with real women. Pictures of naked women have been around since the invention of the camera, but pornography can be exploitive to both men and women. For men, it can become exploitive in the money they pay for the pornography, it can be addictive to have sex with a household appliance (the computer) instead of their wife, and it can be dangerous when it creates unrealistic expectations or the illusions become an obsession.

Danger Signs of Masturbation and/or Pornography

- If your masturbation activities hurt you in any way, such as rubbing skin raw or to the point of bleeding, it's too much. Stop injuring yourself immediately.

- If your sexual activities interrupt with your doing schoolwork, being with friends, or family life, you might have a problem.

- Are you dependent on looking at porn to get excited or aroused? (You can't masturbate or get an erection without it?)

- Do you feel compelled (like you have to do it or you'll feel upset) to masturbate or look at porn?

- Would you rather masturbate and look at porn than do anything else? Ever?

- Do you feel like you "can't stop?"

If you are having any of these danger signs, then get rid of your computer files or magazines now, and stop masturbating for at least a couple of weeks to months. If you are unable to stop or you continue to constantly obsessing about masturbation or pornography, you need to talk to a counselor or sex therapist about your compulsive behavior.

SHARED MASTURBATION

Many guys get together with other guys and masturbate in front of each other, especially before high school age. Some boys report another boy "showed him how." Sometimes it is one on one, with just two guys and sometimes it is a group of guys masturbating. Sometimes these get togethers are called "circle jerks," where guys sit around and masturbate in front of each other, or it might be called a "sausage party." Sometimes it is like a contest, who can shoot the farthest or the fastest? Or, it's a secretive forbidden activity to do that is done in someone's basement or a fort in the woods. For a lot of guys, this is their first sexual experience with another person, even when you are not directly touching each other.

It is estimated about half of men report masturbating in front of another guy at least once in their sexual life, typically when they were very young, around middle school age. Sometimes guys feel very ashamed and worried about these secret masturbation meetings, or that something just kind of "happened." The biggest worry is: *Does this mean I'm gay?* No, half of men are not gay, so this does not mean you are gay. The other worry is, "I'm scared that it felt good and I was with a bunch of guys!" Don't be too worried about have good sexual feelings, even though you are in front of another guy. Your body's sexual wiring doesn't know if you are alone or in front of someone else, or if it is a girl or a guy. You body will often respond to sexual touch, if it is touched sexually. See Chapter Three: Same-Sex Sex, if you are worried about being gay. On the other hand, if you have no interest in doing this, even though it is the "secret, back in the woods, cool neighborhood boys," who are doing this, don't do it if you don't want to! Don't let anyone tease you into doing something you don't want to do, and don't do that to anyone else, either!

By the way, "sausage parties," are, by definition, a guy thing. Girls rarely masturbate in front of each other, and quite frankly, they just don't see the point in why guys would do it.

WET DREAMS

Guys have "nocturnal emissions" or wet dreams, which are ejaculations of semen during your sleep. "Wet dreams," or as they are technically called, "nocturnal emissions," literally means emitting a fluid at night. Wet dreams start happening to guys when they go through puberty. You will just wake up in the morning and have stickiness and wetness on your penis (and/or bedding) from the fluid of ejaculation. According to the good old sex researchers, almost all guys will have this happen on an occasional basis, and it is "normal." As guys begin to masturbate or have other sexual outlets for ejaculation, after they begin to become sexually active, wet dreams are less frequent or non-existent.

The first time or two after this happens, some guys get scared, they don't understand what happens, and might even wonder if they did something wrong, or if they have cancer and are going to die. Wet dreams are a normal way for your body to have a sexual release. Try to understand, accept it and think of it positively, like this: Wow! What a great thing! It's like freebie sex in your sleep! Maybe you're having an erotic dream about the girl next to you in science class, and the next thing you know, you are half awake, feeling warm inside, wet outside, and breathing deeply. Without the hassle of relationships, finding privacy, masturbation, or anything, your body gets sexually aroused, sometimes just biologically or sometimes through a dream, and gives you an orgasm!

THE SPORTS PHYSICAL

Most guys have a sports physical in middle school or high school, for any kind of sports involvement, like football, swimming or soccer. The sports physical includes the usual health tests for blood pressure, heart problems, etc . . . but it also includes a doctor checking for a hernia, which involves examining your genitals. For most guys, this is the first time someone else, since you had your diapers changed, is going to touch your genitals. During a sports physical, the doctor will check you for a hernia (a break in a muscle wall) by reaching and touching you under your testicle, then asking you to "cough," while he feels your muscle movement. Sure, this is a 'normal' medical exam, to determine if you are healthy enough to play sports, but in reality, the doctor will touch your testicles and often your penis is touched or brushed against during this exam.

A lot of guys are secretly afraid of this first sports physical or first sexual examination. By the time you have this exam, it is likely that you've already been touching yourself, and have been masturbating—secretly. A lot of guys are scared that they are going to have a erection and feel very embarrassed, when they are touched. It is true that when you are touched, your body is wired for sexual response, and you may, in fact, get an erection; however, most guys never do. You are in a medical situation, that might last 15 seconds, and you aren't likely to have a sexual response in your doctor's office. Don't worry, the likelihood of getting an erection in this situation has the same odds as being struck by a car: it isn't likely to happen. Even if it does, don't worry about it: it isn't the first erection your doctor has seen is their life. The bottom line is this: don't be scared, it will be over quickly, and no one is going to guess (or ask) that you've been masturbating!

ATTRACTIONS AND AFFECTION

Sharing affection is how people share their feelings of attraction. Most teens have crushes and feelings of attraction toward others. However, many teens, especially guys, are shy about sharing affection. Our society and our families sometimes teach us to be awkward or ashamed about it. Often our families attitudes and behavior toward affection and touch influences how teens and adults feel about affection. Affection is very important to sexuality, especially when it comes to having relationships with girls.

George's Story

George's parents were the "touchy-feely" types. Basically, they were

overgrown hippies from the 70's (George was named after one of the Beatles). His parents were the type who thought that is was healthy and normal to kiss in front of their kids, hug, lie on the couch together, talk about sex, and even sleep in late on the weekends for "alone time."

George felt very embarrassed by his parents. He thought it was pretty gross that they would lie next to each other on the couch and laugh and flirt.

George wanted to tell them to "get a room." Unfortunately, their room was at the end of the hall from his room.

George would ask them to "act normal" when his friends came over, which meant he wanted them to put on stony faces, sit 25 yards away from each other, and not even think about mentioning sex topics. Embarrassingly, his parents were very open and sex wasn't a taboo subject. Once they even about talked about condom use when George's friends came over for pizza.

Basically, George felt humiliated and afraid of his parents embarrassing him, especially in front of his friends. He avoided talking to his parents about any subjects of girls, not to mention sex!

When George was a senior in high school, his best friends' girlfriend was afraid she might be pregnant. It was George's dad who went to the drug store to get the pregnancy test.

When George's girlfriend's best girlfriend got dumped by a guy she had casual sex with and she was ashamed and afraid she might have an STD, she turned to George, and George's mom took her to the doctor.

When George was a freshman in college, he fell in love. He found out he too, was comfortable, and liked hanging out with his girlfriend, talking, laughing, hugging, and flirting . . . on the couch.

After a few years, George realized that his parents taught him to be a person who was understanding and open to people and to affection. By the time he finished college, George learned he, too,

**was comfortable with touching and sexuality, and he stopped being
so embarrassed. Only then did he embraced his parents, and himself, for who he became.**

Guys and girls learn to be "touchy-feely" or avoid touch from
the role models they have with their parents. If you grew up being hugged, kissed, and physically affectionate, you are much more
likely to feel comfortable with affection. If you didn't have this, affection might feel uncomfortable or even unwanted by you.

Even though it might be weird to you now, if your mom wants to
kiss you good-night or hug you good-bye, it is just her way of showing
you affection. A lot of teenage guys withdraw from their moms and
their dads and think it makes them more of a man to reject physical
affection. Many teenage guys think they are too old for a loving kiss
or a hug goodnight. Don't be so afraid or think you are less of a guy
to give your mom or dad a hug, or say you love them . . . *even if it is
not in front of your friends.* All people need hugs and touch!

When you become more confident with yourself and your own
sexuality, and more mature, you will be able to feel more comfortable with affection, with your family, your friends, or your girlfriends.
Attractions and affection toward other people are natural. Learning
how to feel attraction, accept it and express it positively is what you
need in order to grow into a loving man.

CRUSHES, ATTRACTIONS, AND ERECTIONS

By the time you are 12 or 13, you are likely to experience crushes,
attractions, and erections. Crushes, attractions and erections pop up
when you least expect them or want them to happen. And they can
be very embarrassing. And guys usually don't know what to do about
them.

Red's Story

Red was in 8th grade when he had his first experience with an unwanted, untimely erection. He was in Mrs. Connelly's 5th period math class, where he had an eye on Courtney Kemberly, whom he'd had a crush on since 4th grade. Courtney was called to the front of the class to do a homework problem in the front of the room. She was wearing a new pair of tight, hot, black corduroy pants, and a tight pink sweater. Red noticed. He began to watch Courtney's body and forget about the math problem and think about what it would be like to see Courtney naked.

Then, the bell rang.

Red was suddenly stunned and awoke from his sexual fantasy.

Then, Red realized that he had a full erection. He froze. He couldn't move. He couldn't get up. In a flash of a moment, he suddenly felt flushed red with embarrassment and didn't want to stand up, for fear that someone, especially Courtney, would notice that he had a huge erection.

Time seemed to freeze and everyone was moving in slow motion. People were laughing. People were moving. Everyone seemed to be staring at him. Red feared the worst: that they all noticed he had an erection.

What they all noticed is that Red didn't move when the bell rang. He just sat there, like a deer caught in the headlights, frozen in time and not getting up to get to his next class.

Red finally gathered his book and notebook and put it into his bookbag and jumped out of his seat, positioning his bookbag in front of his body. He quickly left his desk and the room and went on to his next class.

On the way, one of Red's best friends, Jack, ran up beside him and said, "Red, no one noticed your boner over Courtney. Stop acting like a freak and keep walking." Red turned and stared at his friend, as if his whole secret crushing world was exposed. Red became

mute with embarrassment. Jack was one of the coolest friends—and the oldest—in his group of friends. Then Jack said, "Hey, just shut up—at least they know you're not gay!" And Red laughed. And Jack laughed. And they made it to the next class together.

For guys, having unexpected erections is a part of life, yet, often an embarrassing experience when you are a teenager. It's normal to have attractions and to crush on girls, as young as in elementary school. But, when you're a teenager, you will begin to experience a sexual response to attractions. Sadly, most guys feel ashamed and want to hide—quickly. Dealing with it is a part of life.

Dealing with it means different things in different situations. If you are in a classroom or public situation, try to cover yourself with a book, bookbag, chair or other large object to avoid the obvious. If someone notices, whether in public or private, your best bet is to avoid direct contact, and if you can't learn to laugh it off in the moment, learn to accept attractions as involuntary, as normal and be easy on yourself. Even a girl will laugh *with* you, if you don't shame yourself and you can laugh at your own humanness. After all, girls have their own sexuality issues, when it comes to the beginning of sex.

153

GIRLS. PERIOD.

You saw the movie (in 4th or 5th grade): now here's the sequel on what guys need to know about girls and . . . periods. Beyond the talk about fallopian tubes and ovaries and menstruation, guys need to know a few things about girls and their monthly cycle. Just like guys have changes with puberty, including body changes, attractions, masturbation, crushes, and erections, as you know, girls have changes, too. Since virgin sex includes having sex with girls: Basically, you've got to learn to deal with their changes and this includes periods.

The Beginning of Sex

Evan's Story

Evan was in the 3rd grade, when he asked his mom about tampons. He had seen the box of white paper wrapped "things" under the bathroom counter. Innocently, he asked his what they were. His mom told him, "They're tampons." Evan asked, "What are tampons?" His mother answered, "They're for grown up girls." Evan was a curious child and asked his mom again, "Yes, but what are they for?" His mom answered, "I told you, they're for girls, for when they grow up." That answer wouldn't do and Evan kept asking questions, "Ok, mommy, but why? What are they for?" His mother answered him, "You don't want to know, I'll explain it when you grow up." Evan wasn't satisfied and he kept pressing his mom for an answer, "Yes, I do want to know, just tell me, what are they for?" His mother told him again, emphatically, "EVAN, NO you DON'T want to know, I'll tell you when you're older." Evan wouldn't take no for an answer and demanded that his mother give him an explanation, "MOM! I want to know! Tell me, I'm a big boy, tell me, I want to know what they are for!"

Exasperated, she began thinking that maybe this very intelligent, curious, and inquisitive 8-year-old, who thought he knew everything, *was* old enough. After all, thanks to his much older stinker stepbrother, Evan already knew about sex: He learned about the "penis and vagina thing" when he was 6. Or maybe his mom wanted to teach Evan a lesson that sometimes when a mom says no, she has a very good reason and sometimes little boys shouldn't be so demanding. So, Evan's mom told him the whole story of girls and periods and babies. After her careful explanation about menstruation and bleeding and the use of tampons, Evan bowed his sweet, little 8-year-old head, got a disgusting look on his face and said, "I didn't want to know."

The truth is that most young guys are grossed out by the idea or thought or conversation about girls' periods. Just because you're uncomfortable, don't just skip this section and run. A lot of guys will take their discomfort and turn it into making jokes, or even teasing and humiliating girls, saying things like: "what a bitch, she must be on the rag" or "I don't trust anyone who bleeds for 5 days and doesn't die," which is cruel. Sure, guys will joke among themselves, especially when it comes to girls' mood swings (see PMS below); however, being cruel to girls you want to befriend, go out with, and have sex with is a bad idea. Learn to feel secure about talking about menstruation, especially since it happens 20% of a girl's life!

> Learning to be comfortable with periods . . . is a rite of passage for men.

155

Most guys try to avoid the subject, because even with most girls, it's a taboo subject: she can bring it up, you can't. Your job as a guy is to try and help girls feel comfortable talking about it when the subject arises. Don't make nasty jokes and demeaning comments, and help out when there is a problem. It will help if *you* learn to feel comfortable with the subject, to treat periods as perfectly normal, and see it as a wonderful, healthy body function.

What you need to know . . .

First, all girls are different. Some girls are very open about their periods or "that time of the month," and many are very shy and embarrassed. For girls, their period, at least in the beginning, is as embarrassing to them as it is for guys to getting erections in untimely situations. Girls are afraid guys will "know" and that they'll be teased and humiliated. The truth is that guys can choose to be very mean,

The Beginning of Sex

or guys can act hero-like toward a girl. Guys can decide to be understanding, supportive, and help girls in difficult situations.

Periodic Period Problems . . . and Solutions

- Her period starts and she doesn't have any tampons or pads with her . . . drive her home and get a fresh supply.

- She has an "accident" and she needs to go home immediately and discreetly change her clothes. An accident means she has blood or a stain on her pants or skirt. Don't freak out . . . just take her home to change.

- Buy tampons or pads. At some point in your younger or older adult life, you will be asked to go the store and buy them for her. Yes . . . you will need to do it. Hint: Find out exactly what type she uses. Better yet, have her write it down or bring the empty box: there are many different brands and sizes.

- You're making out and she tells you she's on her period: Usually this means she doesn't want to have sexual touch. Assume . . . stop! For most girls and women, sex is off-limits during their period, yet, some girls, if they aren't cramping or in pain, don't care. Don't assume . . . ASK!

- Cramps: Most girls have mild to severe cramping and even nausea and vomiting during their periods. Cramping is abdominal pain, and might include back pain and it is real. Be understanding that she might need to rest, be less physically active, or even take medication, if it is severe.

PMS

PMS is short for pre-menstrual syndrome. Many women have mood swings just prior to their period. These can range from mild, with irritability and crankiness for a day, to severe, with yelling and depression for 2 weeks prior to her period. Most girls get bloating, meaning they retain water and feel fat, have breast tenderness, feel tired, and get the blues for a day or two. Most girls don't want to admit they are cranky and they most certainly do not want you to point it out and tell them that they "must be getting their period," even if they are. Some girls have a very easy time with periods and have almost no PMS or other symptoms, like cramping or fatigue, but most have at least mild symptoms some of the time.

The best advice is to be understanding and lay low. Fly below radar: don't start any fights, try to ignore the irritability, be kind and caring, and don't take it personally. After a girl begins her period, that is, when she begins to bleed, her PMS symptoms will subside; however, then the cramping will begin for a few days. If your girlfriend has severe symptoms on a regular basis, you will need to talk to her about it, so you can understand how her periods affect her. Wait until after her period is over to discuss it, so the two of you can be more rational. For severe symptoms, medical treatment is available and helpful.

THE END OF THE BEGINNING OF SEX

Now that you know the beginning of sex, for girls and for guys . . . you are ready to move on to learning more about the basics of sex. So, we'll move on to "definitions," the foundation of sexual information, or the sexual dictionary, to give you more guidance on Virgin Sex.

SIX

REAL SEX ED: THE SEXUAL DICTIONARY FOR GUYS

Most guys, by the time they reach 15, think they know everything there is to know about sex. If you're a typical guy, you think your parents are clueless because you know they think you don't know everything you think you really do know about sex. Yet, as smart, educated, Internet literate, or experienced as you may think you are about sex, every guy can use some real sex ed. Amazingly, even 40 year old doctors that I see in sex therapy always learn things they thought they knew, and they wish they'd known sooner about sex. Now, you're going to know what you need to know now!

WHAT IS SEX?

If you've reached the age of reading, puberty, or whatever the age your parents feels is appropriate to give you this book, and you don't know what sex is, you must have been living on a different planet than Earth. Or, you don't own a T.V., radio, or a computer and you don't attend school or talk to other human beings. Yet, even if you know the basics, about the penis-vagina definition of sex, you will want to know about the secrets of sex with girls. You will need to learn the real truth about sexual basics first, not just the bits and pieces of information you may have picked up and learned from your parents, friends, school sex ed, or even the Internet. In this chapter, you can learn about sexual definitions, the foundations of sex, including the basics of the way sex works, so you can put these pieces together and be ready for a sexual relationship, which is often a mystery to guys (and men).

To unravel the mystery, you need to start with clues. Clues start with definitions, which are the building blocks of information. This chapter is a "dictionary," so to speak, of sexual behaviors. Included are many kinds of words and phrases for sexual behaviors, as well as some black and latino slang names for sex and sexual body parts. Your sexuality may include some or none or all of these behaviors, or they may occur now or at some time in the future, depending on how you choose to express your sexuality. Yet, to begin with sex, having the right language, the right words, and knowing what they mean, will give you the basics of sexual knowledge. Now that you know that you are a sexual being from birth (from Chapter Five), you will want to know the various ways that people describe and express their sexuality.

SEXUAL EXPRESSIONS

Being sexual is much more than sexual intercourse. Sexual expressions can vary from having sexual fantasies to sexual attractions to touching in non-sexual ways to self touch to kissing and hugging to wanting to share your feelings with another person with sexual touch.

What most people mean by "losing your virginity" is generally accepted to mean having sexual intercourse, where a man's erect penis enters a woman's vagina and moves in and out in a way that can or may be pleasurable to both people. Truthfully, a lot of teenagers and young people are virgins who have nevertheless had a lot of sexual experiences, but they have not had sexual intercourse and so their virginity is technically intact. Some guys and girls enjoy sex by themselves, through masturbation. Many girls and guys enjoy having intimate physical experiences, including kissing and hugging, or they enjoy simply sharing their loving feelings without having any sexual contact. Other teens express their loving feelings through kissing, touching, and sexual touching without having sexual intercourse. Really, how people express their sexuality is very personal, very private, and it is only limited by the human imagination. This chapter will discuss the many different ways to express sexuality so that you can start to find the right way for you to express your sexuality.

SEXUAL PARTS . . . SEXUAL WORDS

First, learn about the basics of your body and her body. You should know the names and locations of sexual parts, so when you first see a girl naked, you will have some idea what you are looking at and touching. Even if you have seen a girl naked, or have had sex before, every girl is different. Not all girls are alike. Even if you know something about one girl, it might not work on the next girl. Different girls require different things. One of the joys of being close to someone, is to learn. You don't start learning about sex by having sexual intercourse. You start by talking and then by touching and trying out different things to see how you and she feel, then starting all over again. Unless you've been with someone, you don't know them. With a girl, even if you have physically touched or even sexually played or explored with her before, girls, unlike guys, change how they feel, what they want, and how they like it, sometimes on a daily basis, depending on how they feel at the time. Keep in mind, when you are learning and exploring about sex, that all sexual touch requires sexual permission.

Remember: When it comes to touching, you must always have permission from a girl. Ask, then touch.

Chapter Eight will discuss in detail the three stages of sex, the first being talking and listening. For now, learning the different sexual parts and how they work and respond, is the first part of your real sex ed and the beginning of virgin sex.

SEXUAL SLANG

All of the words below are used for describing sexual parts and sexual behavior. Some of the words more commonly used by African-Americans or Hispanics are listed, too. Of course, every different geographical area has it's own slang, and most importantly, learn what is acceptable to use and say in your town. Of course, you guys need to know that not all of these words are acceptable to girls to be used in everyday conversation. In fact, using some of them might disgust people and cause you to lose potential friendships or relationships. Use your head.

> The use of slang words can be very acceptable in some places, with some people, but be highly emotionally charged in other situations.

Sample Cautions of Slang Use

- Very few guys refer to their penis as "their penis," unless maybe they are talking to their doctor (or sex therapist), and much more commonly call it "their dick," or maybe, "my cock." If you're a guy and you're talking to guys about your dick and you keep calling it "my penis," you're going to look like a moron and nerd.

- Some girls can use and like the word "pussy," but a lot of girls are uncomfortable with that and would rather use the word, "vagina," or "coochie."

- A guy who uses the phrase, "give me some head," with a girl to ask for oral sex, (unless they've been together a long time and they can joke with each other, but maybe not even then) sounds like a degrading demand, not a way to get lucky with the ladies.

- Using the word "cunt" is highly offensive and considered very nasty to a lot of girls and women. For some people, this is the ultimate curse word, way beyond using the "F" word.

GIRL PARTS

The external genital organs of the female are collectively known as the vulva. Most people incorrectly refer to a girls physical anatomy as "her vagina," which is incorrect. Calling the vulva a vagina is like calling a face "the throat." The vulva includes the labia majora and labia minora or the "large" and "small" lips, the clitoris, the clitoral hood, the urethra, the anus, and the vagina, which is actually an internal, not external structure.

Words for Vagina

- Va-va
- Cunt
- Hole
- Box
- Love canal
- Love tunnel

Words for Vulva

- Beaver
- Twat

- Pussy
- Snatch
- Cooter
- Coochie

Words for Breasts

- Tits or titties
- Boobs
- Hooters
- Knockers
- Jugs
- Headlights (refers to erect nipples showing)
- Ta-tas
- Tacos (Hispanic)

163

Words for Clitoris

- Clit
- Magic button
- Hot spot

Girl Touch

The most important thing to know about sexual touch with a girl is that girls don't like to start touching with direct sexual touch. Guys fantasize about having their crotch grabbed, having someone rip their pants off them, then going directly for sexual contact. Girls do not like this at all. Women do like it. This is called groping, when guys grab at a girl's breasts, buttocks, or crotch, and it is a turn-off.

Groping is a sexual turn-off for girls!

Learning to touch, in a non-sexual way, is a basic way of physically connecting with someone you like. Girls like to have touch start and proceed slowly. Girls need to feel comfortable with non-sexual touch before they will want to go any further with you in a physical way. This is true whether you are a virgin and want to have sex for the first time or whether you are 50 years old and have been married forever. Learn to have safe, non-sexual touch to connect first, before you move on to sexual touching.

The Safe Touch Zones

- The "Free Touch Zone": Touching on the arm, from the shoulder to the hand is a free touch zone, meaning anyone can touch someone's arms or hands to give them a pat or touch of reassurance, without having to have permission to touch first. If a girl responds positively with your touching her in the free zone, you can move on to further touch.
- Hands: Holding and touching hands. Gently stroking a girl's hand can be very intimate, as well as exciting to a girl.
- Head and hair: Stroking or playing with hair gently with your fingers
- Face: Gentle touching of the sides of a girl's face, especially before kissing is very intimate, non-sexual touching. Using eye to eye contact creates even greater emotional intimacy.
- Mouth: Kissing, lightly or French kissing (maybe).
- Neck: Touching and kissing the back of the neck is erotic to some girls.
- Shoulders, neck, and back: Rubbing the shoulders, neck, and upper back are very important skills to learn. Touching and rubbing of the back and shoulders, if you have a good connection, is a great way to warm up to further touch.
- Rubbing feet. A good foot rub is a great way to relax and connect.

The Clitoris

The most important sexual part for girls is often NOT the vagina; it's the clitoris. The clitoris has 9,000 nerve endings and is usually easily responsive to sexual touch. Finding, exploring, and touching the clitoris on a young woman, is very important, prior to having sexual intercourse. Touching the clitoris with your finger, mouth, or tongue, is important before you touch any sexual parts with your penis. Most girls can learn to have sexual pleasure with clitoral touch and stimulation.

Before a girl is ready for intercourse sex, an exploration of her sexual parts is essential. Ideally, a girl should have some personal sexual skills before trying to have sexual intercourse, including finding out what she likes sexually and how she responds to sexual touch and even how to bring herself to orgasm. Many young girls don't know this: they don't have a clue. Most young girls will depend on the guy to make them "feel good," and give them an orgasm.

Even though you, as a guy, may not want to control sex, if a girl knows nothing about herself and sexual touch, it is going to be up to you to give her permission, encouragement, guide her, teach her, and help her learn sexual skills to have sexual pleasure. It is not your responsibility to "give her an orgasm," nor should you insist that she have an orgasm, but before you even think of having sexual intercourse, it is essential for girls to learn about their bodies, what feels good to them, how to have sexual pleasure, and to be aroused enough to be able to have sex without physical discomfort or pain. Learning to be aroused with clitoral stimulation is often a key to pleasurable sex for girls.

GUY PARTS

For an illustration of guy parts . . . look in the mirror. Luckily, you guys have it pretty easy: Your parts are right there in front of you, easy to find and easy to define.

165

Words for Penis

- Dick
- Cock
- Dong
- Schlong
- Wee-wee
- Willy
- Rod
- Wang
- Wiener
- Peter
- Pecker
- Johnson

Words for Testicles

- Balls
- Nuts
- Jewels
- Rocks
- Nuggies

Words for Anus

- Ass
- Asshole
- Butthole

Word for Buttocks

- Butt
- Ass

- Rear end
- Fanny
- Junk in the trunk

TYPES OF SEXUAL BEHAVIORS

Fantasies

Fantasies are one of the first ways that people express their sexuality. Fantasies are your thoughts about sex. One of the great things about fantasies is that they are safe: you can't get someone pregnant, you can't get hurt, you can't get STDs, and you don't have to have anyone's permission to enjoy them! Thinking about sex, and thinking about yourself and other people in a sexual way, is a normal part of being a sexual person. Fantasies may be a way for you to explore how you might feel about a person, place, or sexual situation. You don't have to act on your fantasies, but you can explore your feelings about sex in your own imagination.

Sometimes fantasies may be just thinking about someone you have a huge crush on. You might think about a girl talking to you, and you might rehearse in your mind how you would act. Sometimes fantasies are about someone you know you'll never meet or be with, like a movie star, or maybe the captain of the cheerleading team, if she moves in social circles you don't care to join. Some fantasies involve a certain place you imagine being romantic or sexy, such as the beach or your bedroom.

Fantasies can be a fun way to get turned on. Guys usually have sexual fantasies every day, several times a day, and all of their life. Girls, on the other hand, do not think about sex as much. Girls fantasize (a lot) about a guy liking them or talking to them or holding and kissing them, but some girls never have sexual thoughts or fantasies. With permission and encouragement, girls can have sexual fantasies more often, too. Sexual fantasies can be fun to share or role-play together, when you feel much more comfortable with each other, have excellent sexual communication, and have sexual trust.

Fantasies can become a problem if you can't get sexually excited without thinking about them. If you *only* get turned on by fantasies, and you don't get turned on by real life sexual activities, then you might have a problem. Another problem with fantasies is if you are obsessing about certain things that are very disgusting to you and you can't get them off your mind. If you find yourself being stuck on a fantasy that bothers you and you can't seem to have other sexual feelings that are right for you, you should consider talking to a professional, such as a sex counselor or therapist.

Masturbation

Words for Female Masturbation

- Self-loving
- Self-stimulation
- Self-pleasuring
- Paddling the pink canoe
- Rubbing off
- Combing the clit
- Vibrating off
- Buzzing off
- Self-touching
- Playing with yourself
- Fingering yourself

Words for Male Masturbation

- Jacking off
- Jerking off

- Spanking the monkey
- Choking the chicken
- Bopping the bologna
- Beat the meat
- Flog the hog
- Relieving yourself
- Yanking the plank
- Beating off
- Getting off
- Masturbation
- Self-stimulation
- Self-pleasuring
- Self-loving
- Bobbing the dolphin
- Shining the knob
- Rubbin' the nubbin
- Pounding the mound

Do you notice the big difference in the vocabulary available for guys and girls for sexual parts, and especially masturbation? I took a linguistics class several years ago in college. It was about how language was developed and used in different cultures. I never thought I would ever be able to use any of the knowledge from that class (do you know what I mean?), which was required for college graduation, but what I learned is that when cultures have many words for one thing, that one thing is important and significant in their culture. For example, in most of America, we have one word for snow: snow. Eskimos, apparently, have many words for snow, because it is such an important part of their life and culture. Since men have so many more phrases for masturbation, it's obvious that male masturbation is seen as more important and acceptable in our culture for men.

Words or Phrases for Sexual Behaviors

Words or Phrases People Use for Sex

- Making love
- Sexual intercourse
- Having sex
- Sleeping together
- Fucking
- Sexing
- Screwing
- Banging
- Shagging—A Great Britain term
- Jumping your bones
- Tapping it
- Doing the nasty
- Humping
- Getting a piece of ass
- Getting some
- Doing it
- Boning
- Chopping—"Hey you wanna chop?"
- Cuttin'/cutting—"Can I cut?"
- Slamming—Can I slam?
- Hittin' it/hit it—Can I hit that?
- Beatin'/beating
- Tapping it
- Can I beat?

Words or Phrases for Oral Sex on a Girl

- Cunnilingus
- Oral sex

- Eating pussy
- Eating her out
- Going down on her
- Muff diving
- Eating at the "Y"
- Carpet munching

Words or Phrases for Oral Sex on a Guy

- Fellatio
- Oral sex
- Blow job
- BJ
- Sucking him off
- Giving Head
- Knowledge
- Neck

Words or Phrases for Casual Sex

- Friends with benefits
- Sportsexing
- Bed buddies
- Sportsfucking
- Fuck buddies
- Playing the field

Casual sex is a term used when people have sex outside a committed relationship, such as marriage, engagement, or a monogamous relationship. A monogamous relationship means that two people are committed to each other and have no other sexual partners. Whether or not you have such a sexual arrangement will depend on your own moral associations with uncommitted sex and your comfort level with such behavior. Many people, especially girls and people whose religious values are important to them, regret casual sex. Sex within a caring relationship enhances a sexual experience for most people, and monogamous sex is much safer sex, considering STDs and pregnancy. Yet, the truth is that many guys desire to have sex outside of relationships in order to have sexual closeness without the responsibilities that accompany a deeper relationship. You will have to consider these things for yourself relative to your own conditions for sex.

SEXUAL RESPONSE AND ORGASMS

As stated previously, our bodies are wired for sex, and as you get more and more excited, or aroused, and then engage in sexual acts and have a sexual release your body will go through a series of physical responses to sex, called the sexual response cycle. There are four basic stages of sexual response: (1) sexual desire, (2) sexual arousal, (3) orgasm, and (4) relaxation, each of which will be described below. (Masters & Johnson, 1966) Both men and women experience the stages of sexual response.

Each person is different and every situation is different, and you will not go through the whole cycle of responses every time you think about or have sex. Sometimes you might have a lot of excitement but not really get physically aroused or even come close to having an orgasm. At another time, you might not even feel so excited but an orgasm just seems to happen. The sexual response cycle is a process that each person experiences uniquely, but it is important to understand and learn what may happen when you get sexually excited in order to be prepared for sexual situations and your body's response to them. Most guys and girls know what it feels like to get sexually excited, but sexual responses range from feeling sexual desire to feeling physically turned on to having an orgasm or climax. It is important for guys to be prepared for what happens to a man and woman's body in each stage.

Sexual Desire

The first stage of sexual response is sexual desire. Sexual desire is thinking about sex or the feeling of wanting sexual touch, by yourself or with a partner. For many people, especially for teen guys, it is called "being horny."

For most guys, sexual desire is something that happens without any kind of sexual stimulation, such as visual stimulation, like looking at someone you think is hot or having sexual touch. As you know, the truth is, guys think about sex a lot. Sexual desire for guys comes naturally, it is hormonal, and it is an everyday thing.

For girls, sexual desire can happen without any sexual thoughts or stimulation, but usually there is some kind of trigger or sexual stimulation that makes them think about sex. For girls, they might be thinking about something sexy or look at someone who turns them on, and they may feel sexual excitement or desire as a result.

> For some girls, they do not feel sexual desire or the wanting of sex, until after they feel sexual touch and physical excitement

This is a very important difference in men and women. Men need to realize that a lot of women don't just get horny, like guys do. Girls and women need a transition from thinking about everyday life to thoughts about sex. Usually, emotional intimacy, which is talking and spending time together with someone they like, and non-sexual touch (see safe sexual touching, above) are ways for girls to make that transition and feel sexual desire. For some girls, they don't even think about sex or feel horny until they are in a physically intimate situation. For example, some girls don't think about sex until after they are kissing or after making out or after they experience physical touch.

Some girls do have strong sexual desires. Sometimes these are real physical desires like guys have, and girls will go after guys and initiate sex. Some girls will use sex, or manipulate guys with sex, to get what they want: emotional closeness. In either case, girls can be very aggressive with sex, and want sex, too. Guys need to know that girls often have emotional desires first: to want to be with a guy, have a boyfriend, and desire to be talk to and be close to a special person.

Remember Sammy, from Chapter One and Chapter Two? Sammy felt pressured by his first girlfriend to have sex, then got dumped by her. Then, after they'd broken up, over the next year, Sammy had at least 7 times when a girl offered to give him oral sex if he would be their boyfriend or even for no reason at all! Sammy felt somewhat intimidated by so many aggressive girls coming after him and putting sexual demands on him. At several times (seven, to be exact, in one year), Sammy had girls offering him oral sex, if he would be their boyfriend. Was this sexual desire on the girl's part or their desire to have an emotional connection and use sex to manipulate Sammy? Girls do have sexual desire, but guys need to watch out for girls' motivations when they are aggressive about sex.

Sexual Arousal

Sexual arousal means feeling sensations of physical excitement or being "turned on." Physical sexual arousal shows for guys when they get an erection. Guys have erections every 90 minutes, from birth and for the rest of their lives, to some extent, whether they are conscious of sexual desire or not. Guys know when they are physically aroused, because their erection is right there in front of them. Girls are different. Girls get sexually aroused or get lubricated every 90 minutes, too, but often, they are not aware of it.

For girls, sexual excitement shows when their vagina gets lubricated or "wet." When girls get aroused, their vaginas get moist and their vaginas expand: the vaginal walls get thicker and expand in length, making the penetration of a finger or penis possible. A girl's vagina often expands about 2 inches in length during arousal. The average girl's vagina is 4 inches in length, which means when she is aroused, it expands to 6 inches. The average length of a man's erect penis is also 6 inches in length. So, when a girl is sexually aroused, it allows her to accommodate the average size of a man's penis. If a girl has sex with a guy when she is not physically aroused, when her vaginal length is only 4 inches and his penis length is 6 inches, sexual intercourse will cause sexual pain. With a lack of sexual arousal, a man's penis during sexual thrusting will hit against the woman's cervix (at the end of her vagina) and cause her to feel sexual discomfort or pain. Hence, it is very, very important that a woman be sexual aroused to be able to have enjoyable sex.

Usually, if you are attracted to someone, you will begin to get sexually aroused just from talking and being with each other. Most girls will get physically aroused with touch that doesn't include sexual areas, including kissing, hugging, and caressing of the face, hair, arms, legs, and body. Sometimes physical arousal happens from visual stimulation or just looking at your partner's body. Physical arousal also usually happens with touching of the sexual areas: the breasts, buttocks, clitoris, vulva, or vagina, but especially with clitoral stimulation. Sometimes girls can feel when they get aroused, but a lot of girls don't know if they're "wet" unless their underwear is wet or they feel themselves with their fingers. Likewise, a guy can know if a girl is aroused by feeling if she is lubricated or wet with his finger or mouth, prior to having sexual intercourse.

Sources of Sexual Arousal

- Touch
- Smell
- Sight

- Sound
- Kissing
- Music
- Sexy movies
- A deep emotional connection
- Sexual fantasies

Some girls are not able to have physical sexual arousal. That is, they do not feel excited, they do not get wet and lubricated, and they are unable to have an orgasm. Some women do have orgasms without lubrication, but that is uncommon in younger women. A number of factors may cause a lack of sexual excitement, but a lack of arousal usually means that a girl is not prepared for vaginal penetration, emotionally and/or physically. There are many reasons for a lack of physical arousal. The most common are:

- She may be too nervous to get relaxed and aroused for sex
- She may have conflicts with her sexual values
- She may have experienced sexual trauma in her past
- She may not be ready for anything sexual yet
- She may not have any emotional feelings for you that lead to physical arousal
- Her mind says yes, but her body says no

Orgasm

The next stage of sexual response is the orgasm. For many teenage guys, an orgasm happens to them or they experience orgasm through some type of self stimulation or masturbation. As discussed in Chapter Five, guys often have "wet dreams" or nocturnal emissions. Also, most guys experience orgasm through rubbing, touching, dry humping, or masturbation that brings them to orgasm and they experience orgasm or ejaculation. The biggest change that boys experience is when they cross the line to becoming "comers," or start to ejaculate seminal fluid when they have an orgasm. Most boys experience this between the ages of 11–14.

For girls, orgasms are something that they have to figure out, or make happen to them. Unlike guys, who have one type of orgasm that generally peaks with ejaculation, with girls it is generally accepted that there are two different types of orgasms: clitoral and vaginal. A clitoral orgasm is a peak of sexual arousal that usually happens following touching, rubbing, or stimulation of the clitoris. The second type of orgasm is a vaginal orgasm, which results from penetration and stimulation inside of the vagina with a penis or a finger or a dildo.

Defining an "orgasm" for girls is very different than it is for guys, as it is experienced very differently among women. With guys, they generally share similar experiences with orgasm being associated with ejaculation. With women, physically, an orgasm is a peak of sexual excitement and muscle tension, with a series of muscle contractions, including the contraction of the muscles in their uterus, though the vagina, clitoris, and pelvic regions, and a release of those muscles. Some women report feeling like fireworks go off and explosions shoot through their bodies. Other women report feeling their muscles tense and release and that the experience was "OK." However, orgasm usually feels very good, and it can be very intense. Guys know when they come, girls sometimes don't know when they have an orgasm, at least when they first experiment with sex.

Girls may have orgasms from very young ages, as early as 3 or 4, but most women do not report experiencing orgasms until after puberty. Not all women have orgasms. Approximately 78% of women under 30 have clitoral orgasms, but with instruction, practice, and sometimes the use of a vibrator almost all women can have clitoral orgasms. Fewer women experience vaginal orgasms than clitoral orgasms. About 30% of women have them all the time, 30% of women have them some of the time, and the rest of women don't experience the sensation at all. Again, with practice and guidance, many women can have vaginal orgasms, too. Some women must have stimulation of the clitoris, through body or hand rubbing during intercourse, so that they can have an orgasm with vaginal penetration, but the orgasm comes from clitoral stimulation. Some women have orgasms only by themselves and not with a partner; that is, they may have orgasms through masturbation, but not with a sexual partner. Many women do not have orgasms all the time, with every sexual experience.

Sadly, most teenage girls do not have orgasms with their male partners. Usually, this is from a lack of experience: girls not knowing how to have an orgasm and boys not knowing how to give them one. This situation is a result of girls not knowing their own bodies or of girls not using their sexual voice to tell their partners what they want. Sometimes, this is also a result of guys not knowing or caring about what they are doing with regard to a girl's needs. Guys, this needs to change, and *you* need to be the ones to change it. If a girl is not getting anything out of sex, this is called bad sex!

It is really not decided in sex research circles why some women have vaginal orgasms and others don't. Many researchers believe that women have a "G-spot," or the Grafenberg spot, which is a place about two inches inside of the vagina on the belly button side that causes intense vaginal orgasms when it is stimulated by a finger, dildo, or penis. Finding and stimulating the "G-spot," works for many women to have orgasms during sexual penetration, and many of the 50% of women who do not have vaginal orgasms at all can learn.

Some women have orgasms without any physical touch at all. They can "think off." They can have an orgasm simply through sexual fantasy. Some women have orgasms without genital touch, such as via the touching of their nipples. Women can also have orgasms from anal sex. Many women have the ability to have more than one orgasm, or multiple orgasms.

Ejaculation

Premature Male Ejaculation

Premature ejaculation is when a guy ejaculates or comes before he wants to during sex. Believe it or not, one out of three guys has a problem with premature ejaculation in his lifetime, usually as a young man. Clinically, the definition of premature ejaculation or rapid ejaculation is lasting less than one minute, meaning a guy comes within one minute from the beginning of sexual thrusting during intercourse.

Premature ejaculation is the most common sexual problem for guys. Having ejaculatory control takes time, patience, and sometimes practice to learn. The common sexual myth is that a guy should try to think of other things besides sex, such as baseball statistics, to keep his mind off his sexual excitement and keep himself from coming. Actually, the solution to premature ejaculation is exactly the opposite. To learn ejaculatory control, a guy needs to think and feel more about sex and learn to experience more intense sexual arousal to delay the "arousal phase" (as described above) of sexual arousal, in order to delay ejaculation. Often, one of the biggest problems with premature ejaculation is simply being nervous about sex. Guys need to learn to relax, focus on the pleasure of sex, rather than worry about their sexual performance and learn to handle sexual arousal more intensely, one step at a time.

Female Ejaculation

Some women ejaculate fluid from the urethra (where urine comes out) during orgasm. Some researchers have found that this occurs when the G-spot is stimulated. This fluid has been found not to be urine but a fluid unique to intense sexual pleasuring. It is normal, just like a man's ejaculation during intercourse is normal. Generally, during sex, wetness from lubrication and ejaculation will leave a "wet spot" on the bed or surface upon which people have sexual acts. This wet spot might be a few inches in diameter or length. With female ejaculation, the amount of fluid ejaculated is increased, and the wet spot can be as large as a foot in diameter.

Relaxation

The fourth stage of sexual response is relaxation. This means that the body relaxes, physically, and returns to a state of normal, or non-sexual arousal. For some people, this means the end of a sexual encounter. However, for some people, they may choose to continue with sexual activity and rerun the sexual cycle again. Both men and women are able to have multiple sexual episodes or sexual cycles in a row or multiple orgasms.

MULTIPLE ORGASMS

Multiple orgasms mean having orgasm one after another. For both sexes this means having maybe two or three orgasms in one sexual encounter. Women are different than men in this way: they can physically have as many orgasms as they would like to have in one sexual encounter: they can have 2, 3, or even maybe fifteen orgasms in one day or more. Multiple orgasms does not mean that a person has more than one orgasm at the same time: it means you have one orgasm after the other. Most women, though, are very sensitive on their clitoris and vulva after having an orgasm. They need to wait a few minutes or so to be able to be sexually aroused again in order to have more than one orgasm. After waiting a few minutes or 15 minutes or so, they are able to enjoy sexual stimulation and arousal and have another orgasm, if they so desire.

Men are usually pretty much done after one or two or at the most a few ejaculations. They simply run out of semen after awhile and have to wait for it to be replenished. Men have a "refractionary period," after ejaculation. This means that most guys, after an orgasm, have to wait a period of time before they are able to have another erection and another ejaculation or orgasm. For young teenage guys, this time period is usually very short, sometimes just a few minutes. As men age, this time period gets longer, up to 24 hours long when they are old.

MORE SEXUAL WORDS

Abstinence: Not engaging in sexual relations, especially sexual intercourse. "Continuous abstinence" means not ever having sex. "Periodic abstinence" means not having sexual intercourse during some periods of time, which is not safe sex.

Anal sex: Stimulation or penetration of the anus.

AIDS: Acquired Immune Deficiency Syndrome, a sexually transmitted disease that causes death.

Bisexuality: Having sexual relationships with both sexes.

Blow jobs: Oral sex. Oral sex on a guy is sucking or licking his penis. Oral sex on a girl is kissing and licking her clitoris.

Clitoris (KLIT-o-ris) or (klit-TOR-is, the pronunciation differs geographically): A small, very sensitive piece of skin located at the top of the vulva, just below the pubic bone. It is more easily found with touch rather than sight because it is small, but very sensitive to touch, often tingling on contact. The sole purpose of the clitoris is for sexual arousal, and it is very important for sexual pleasure.

Clitoral hood: A layer of skin that surrounds the clitoris.

Condom: A rubber, latex, or animal-skin sheath made to cover the penis and prevent pregnancy and reduce the risk of sexually transmitted diseases.

Dildo: A sexual "toy" that is generally made out of plastic or soft or hard rubber that is in the shape of a penis. It is for use in vaginal or anal penetration during sex.

Diaphragm: Birth control device, shaped like a small dome, made out of latex to fit inside the vagina and over the cervix.

Erection: When a guy's penis is hard and stiff.

Ejaculation: When semen comes out of the urinary opening or small hole on the head of the penis.

Foreplay: Any physical touching, including sexual touching, that does not include sexual intercourse.

HIV: Human acquired immunodeficiency virus. This is the virus that many scientists believe causes AIDS. When someone "gets AIDS," they first get the HIV virus. Many people live with HIV for several years before it "turns into" AIDS.

Hymen: A membrane, or layer of skin, that partially covers the inside of the vagina. The hymen is generally opened when a girl loses her virginity, but it can be opened through vigorous athletic activity or tampon use. Slang: "cherry" or "maidenhead."

Monogamy: Both sexual partners having sex only with each other; not having other sexual partners.

Outercourse: A newer term referring to sexual play that does not involve anal or vaginal intercourse.

Semen: The fluid ejaculated when a male has an orgasm.

STDs: Sexually transmitted diseases (see Chapter Seven). STDs are often referred to as STIs, or sexual transmitted infections, which is a preferred politically correct term.

Vibrator: A "sexual toy" that may be in the shape of a dildo, except that is has batteries and vibrates. Or a wand-shaped device that vibrates, usually used for clitoral stimulation; may be plugged in or powered by batteries.

Virgin sex: Sex for the first time. Virgin sex can be any sexual experience, including self-touch, mutual sexual touching, oral sex, and sexual intercourse. Some people think "real sex" is sex that involves sexual intercourse, but the truth is that all sexual acts are a form of sexual behavior and thus virgin sex is the first time you do any of these things. However, you only lose your virginity, technically speaking, when you have sexual intercourse for the first time. Virgin sex should be pure and not dirty or bad or painful. Sex for the first time can be a positive, joyful experience, rather than tainted with pain that sometimes lasts many years.

SEVEN

STDS, SAFER SEX, AND BIRTH CONTROL

Before you consider having sex, seriously consider being safe about sex. One of the biggest concerns that parents have about their children, when it comes to sex, is the fear that their child, that you, will get hurt from sex, by getting a sexually transmitted disease or getting someone pregnant. Two of the biggest sexual mistakes that guys make are not taking precautions against STDs or pregnancy, by not practicing safer sex or using birth control.

> One in four teenagers gets an STD and one in five sexually active teens gets pregnant.

Since 25% of teens get STDs or pregnant or both, parents' worries about STDs and pregnancy are very realistic. Just think about it: if you are sexually active, there is a very real chance that you or someone you have sex with will get an STD or get pregnant. To picture your odds of getting an STD or getting pregnant, especially if you are not responsible and do not practice safer sex, think about you and your closest three friends. If all of you are sexually active as teenagers, at least one of you will get an STD and least one of you will get someone pregnant by the time you are 19. Don't think it can't happen to you or your friends: it will, unless you are willing to learn how to be responsible with sex.

> In fact, if you do not use birth control when you are sexually active, there is a 90% chance you will get someone pregnant within a year!

This chapter is not about scare tactics or lies: it is simply about telling you the truth, to help you learn how to avoid getting hurt by sex and maybe help you help your friends, by choosing abstinence or choosing to practice safer sex. Making sexual choices are not a one time event, they are ongoing choices, chances, situations, and moments that will occur over your entire lifetime. Learn to make good choices early in your sexual life, but even if you make a mistake and get hurt by sex, you can always learn to make better choices for your future.

GETTING BURNED

Obviously, one of the most negative consequences of sex can be acquiring a sexually transmitted disease since you can die from some of them. Sexually transmitted diseases are diseases that are passed from person to person through sexual contact, and specifically, from the exchange of sexual bodily fluids. Sexually transmitted diseases are called "STDs," "VD" for venereal disease, and "STIs" for sexually transmitted infections. Another common slang for STDs is called "getting burned."

This book will provide just a brief overview of STDs for you, since there are lots of other resources on STDs and this is not the major focus of this book. The Internet has many health sites that offer more extensive information on STDs, and you can also find information about STDs at the public library.

Whether you are having sex for the first time or you've had many sexual partners, you want to protect yourself from STDs. STDs can kill you, make you or your sexual partner infertile (you can't have children), or maybe just make your crotch itch like crazy and burn when you urinate!

A lot of times, you can't tell if you have an STD or when someone else has one just by looking at them. Some STDs that are immediately infectious but remain undetectable (you don't know you have it), such as HIV or syphilis, which can be transmitted or given to sexual partners without your knowledge. That's why STDs spread so fast. Once someone is infected with an STD, they can give it to their sexual partner. STDs are spread through close skin-to-skin genital contact or by bodily fluids shared during vaginal, oral, or anal sex, which include blood, semen, and vaginal fluids.

> Every time you have sex with someone, when it comes to STDs, biologically speaking, both of you are having sex with every previous sexual partner you have ever had, every previous sexual partner your sexual partner has had, every previous sexual partner their previous sexual partners have ever had, and so on.

Since there is no way that you can know about everyone's sexual history and sexual health, you need to take care of your own health and protect the future health of those people you care about or love by practicing safe or safer sex. That is why if either of you have engaged in sexually risky behavior, it is best to be tested for STDs to avoid spreading diseases, before you have any sexual contact. It is very important to go to a doctor or even a free clinic to have a medical screening for STDs. Having an STD can have an effect on your whole life, including your health, your future sexual relationships, and your ability to have children. Even if it doesn't seem that important at the moment, being irresponsible now with unsafe sexual practices can affect you for your entire life.

COMMON TYPES OF SEXUALLY TRANSMITTED DISEASES

HIV/AIDS

HIV and AIDS is the most feared STD, because there is no cure. Although people are living longer and better quality lives while living with AIDS, medical treatment is expensive, requiring an extensive routine of many drugs, if you can afford them, and, ultimately, they may not work. Human immunodeficiency virus, also called HIV, is a virus that destroys your immune system. Without an immune system, which protects you from illnesses and diseases, your body can get very sick from ordinary infections, or rare types of infections. People who have HIV can become very ill to the point that they can't fight disease. When the body is very ill from HIV and doesn't have enough healthy cells to fight germs, HIV turns into acquired immune deficiency syndrome, or AIDS. People don't actually die from AIDS, they die from having a weak immune system and getting a disease they can't fight off. You can get HIV in the same way as you get other STDs: through the sharing of bodily fluids during sexual activity. Also, you can also get infected with HIV from having contact with the body fluids, including blood, of someone who has HIV, either from sexual activity or through a cut, tear, or other broken skin opening. HIV can also be passed on to a child during pregnancy or from breast milk. Infections from blood usually happen when needles are shared with intravenous drug use, in blood transfusions, and from even tiny amounts of blood shared during sexual activity. People usually get HIV from sexual intercourse—vaginal or anal—or sharing infected drug needles. All too often, people are really afraid of being around people who have HIV or AIDS and just getting it from everyday contact. HIV isn't like catching a cold: You can't get it from hugging, kissing, breathing the same air, sharing a glass, or just hanging out with someone who has it.

HIV can be avoided by not having intercourse, not using other people's drug needles, and always using protection if you choose to have any sexual contact that involves exchanging body fluids.

Every teen can learn from other teens, experiences and learn to make better choices about sex, especially when it comes to the HIV virus and AIDS. The following letter was found online at a website posting, www.hivaids.webcentral.com.au/text/stories.html, for AIDS/HIV stories.

Anonymous in New York

Well, it all started out when I was 16 years old and I was having unprotected sex with my boyfriend. I didn't think ever this would happen to me, and I don't know why it did. I didn't do anything wrong, it was just a harmless thing as having sex. Well, we went to many parties, and I got drunk, ended up having unprotected sex with about 3 boys or more. I was very stupid. A few weeks later, I got a cold. Well, it started getting worse and worse, I didn't know what was wrong with me. I started feeling very 'out of it.' I thought I was going to die, I could hardly breath! My mother made me go to the doctor. I didn't think anything of it. I just thought I must have caught something very severe. But, I was wrong. The doctor was checking, then he said, "I am going to check your blood." He said "It may be something there." So he did, it took days and days and I think even weeks for the results to come. Well, my mother came to me, it was almost my 17th birthday. So, I thought [it was] something about having my party. But no, she came with the results. She read it all first, she was crying. I was so confused, then I found out I was HIV-positive. I started crying, she didn't know I was having unprotected sex with so many guys. It was just a very bad moment, I wish never happened. It was as if my mother didn't trust me anymore, my mother told my father, then talked [about] if it was 'safe' to tell the whole family. Well, they ended up telling them anyways. Now, that people know I have AIDS, it's as if I am so 'different' from people. No one even looks at me like they used to anymore. I am 20 years old now, so it didn't happen too long ago. It's so bad though, it could have been as simple as having protective sex, as simple as that! I didn't think back then, now I do. And now that I do, no one even comes near me. So, I feel as if no one loves me now. But I know my family does, even if everyone knows the truth, its better that way. I don't want to ruin anyone else's lives, because I ruined mine. So think about this. You should always have protected sex, and trust the people that you do have sex with.

To read more about teens and stories about AIDS, including several stories about AIDS scares and living with AIDS, check out the website above.

Teens get HIV because they have sexual intercourse, usually unprotected sex and have been reckless, sometimes just once, sometimes many times, *and they simply thought it wouldn't happen to them.* It is very easy to get caught up in the notion that everyone is having unprotected sex and they're not getting AIDS and one time or two times or a few times isn't going to matter. The truth is a LOT of teens have unprotected sex, even when they know better, and then they get very scared that they will get HIV or another STD. The fear alone can be life changing, making you worry all the time that you might die or get someone pregnant, or have to live with HIV.

It causes a tremendous amount of guilt and fear and makes your life miserable. Life is much easier to practice safer sex or abstain from sex, at least until you have a partner you really, truly can trust and who is willing to take safer sex seriously.

Every teen reading this book knows about AIDS and has had the subject crammed down your throat by the time you have reached middle school. Still, people like "Anonymous," have unprotected sex, even though they know better, because it just seems to be a part of being a teen, to do impulsive things that you regret later. A lot of teenagers have very similar stories as the one "Anonymous" shares. A lot of teens, both boys and girls, from all kinds of different families and backgrounds, including smart, "straight A" kids who have very bright futures, from black to white to Hispanic and Asian make sexual mistakes. AIDS is definitely an "equal opportunity" disease that only takes one sexual mistake. Some of you guys might be thinking you are having sex with a seemingly nice girl who would, could, never will have sex with anyone else, because they're "good girls." Those good girls make mistakes, too, like "Anonymous in New York."

> The only one who can protect yourself is YOU. AIDS is preventable. Every day you make a sexual choice, you can create a new future or prevent the wrong future for yourself.

Chlamydia

Chlamydia is the most common bacterial STD, infecting one in seven women under 30 years old. Often guys feel no symptoms and they don't know they have it. Symptoms can include itching, burning, painful urination, abdominal pain, and girls have a vaginal discharge that may smell funky. When it is treated with drugs, it causes no lifelong problems. However, if it is untreated, it can cause a lot of damage to a girl's reproductive system and make her infertile, which means she will never be able to have children. Sexually active teens need to be checked regularly for STDs, especially chlamydia, since is it so common and it may cause permanent damage. Even though guys may not become infertile, you can easily give Chlamydia to another girl. Just think: that girl or some girl might be *the* girl with whom you will one day want to have a family, but can't, causing a lot of heartache for the rest of your life.

Genital Herpes

Herpes is a virus, and one out of four adults is infected with it. There is no cure for herpes, although it is not life-threatening. There are two kind of herpes. Type I is common cold sores on the mouth, also known as fever blisters or canker sores. Type I herpes are common, but fairly harmless, except they cause recurrent cold sores at times of stress. The other kind is genital herpes, Type II, which causes painful blisters, sores, or red-rimmed bumps on the penis, vulva, anus, and even on the mouth. Type II herpes can have serious problems for people, including complications for women during pregnancy. What most people don't know, even adults, is that in the last several years, *the two types of herpes are very commonly interchanged.* This means that some people who simply seem to have fever blisters or cold sores on their mouth really have genital herpes on their mouth! As of right now, 30% of oral herpes is actually the genital herpes type, and the rate of oral herpes that is actually genital herpes is increasing every year. So, when someone has what looks like a cold sore on the mouth, it might actually be Type II genital herpes. Oral herpes can be spread by both kissing, and by any oral contact, including touching an open sore and oral sex.

> Herpes is an STD that doesn't go away. Once you have it, you have it for life. You can get it from oral sex or kissing.

Most people do not know that genital herpes can be transmitted from oral-genital contact, meaning that you can get herpes from someone who has what looks like a cold sore, during oral sex! Herpes is very contagious, and spreads from skin-to-skin contact with the blisters or bumps. Because it is so contagious, you must be very careful not to spread the infection to other parts of your body, such as your eyes (you can go blind!), or to other people.

The bad thing about herpes is that it isn't a one-shot deal. Once they have it, many people get recurrent outbreaks for life. Typically, a person may have one or two outbreaks per year, when they are under stress or physically run down. Some people never get a second outbreak, but some people have outbreaks every month! Some people have the disease, but never experience any symptoms, although they can spread it to other people without knowing it. The first herpes outbreak is typically the worst, with painful blisters, pelvic soreness, itching, burning, and even flu-like symptoms. Subsequent outbreaks may only be red bumps, but with itching or burning. Untreated, the sores last about ten days, but with medication, sores begin to disappear in two to four days. Medication can be used every day to control having any outbreaks.

Genital Warts/HPV

Brad's Story

Brad woke up and dragged himself into the shower. He began to wash, but when he reached down to wash his genitals, it hurt! He looked down at his crotch, and his penis has little bumps right on top

of the tip of his dick! Not just one or two, but there were at least 8 or 10 little whitish bumps that he could see and count. He got really scared and tried to scrub them off. It didn't help. It hurt. Then he got on the Internet and started looking up "bumps on your genitals." He learned that he'd either slept with a swarm of insects and got a lot of bug bites or he had herpes or he had genital warts. He was hoping a giant swarm of gnats had come into his bedroom, on the second floor of his parent's house, and ate his crotch alive that night. But, he knew that wasn't it: he was just in denial of what he knew was probably true.

Two weeks earlier, Brad had had sex with an old girlfriend that he hadn't seen for a long time, but they had never had sex before. She was older, and a freshman in college and he was a junior in high school. She was teasing him because he was still a virgin, but not really harshly; nevertheless, Brad felt embarrassed that he was still a virgin. Brad had really, really liked Tara, but they were really young when they were together and they never went all the way. Tara broke up with Brad because she thought he was too young for her, he guessed, because she started going out with older guys. That had always made Brad feel stupid and inferior and awkward, even though he really still liked her for a while, but that only made him feel mad at himself and he moved on. Eventually, they hardly saw each other, until two years later.

They saw each other at a party, really just some friends hanging out at a friend's house. Tara was on the rebound from just breaking up with her boyfriend, who had cheated on her. They started talking and it seemed like no time had passed. They were talking and Tara was crying her eyes out to him over her recent ex, and they felt very close in just one night. Brad had been very sweet and supportive to her over her boyfriend and she felt sorry for him still being a virgin when she wasn't anymore. So, out of mutual pity, more than love, they ended up having sex. He helped her try to get over her ex and she "helped him" lose his virginity. Besides pity, Brad still did have a

STDs, Safer Sex, and Birth Control

lot of feelings for Tara and he had always wanted Tara to be his first, so it seemed like a good idea at the time to Brad to have sex for the first time with her.

Two weeks later, Brad started panicking, as he kept searching the Internet for an answer. Throughout the day, he kept unzipping his pants, checking his groin, and finding the bumps, still sitting there. Finally, Brad decided he had to go to the doctor, to find out what he had. He told his mom he wasn't feeling good and he thought he had the flu. She started looking in the cabinet for some medicine, and got out some mild pain reliever for him. He took it, which didn't help a little bit, because he knew he really needed to go to the doctor and get some different medication. He just couldn't get the courage to tell his mom about the bumps.

Finally, he called his dad. His mom and dad had been divorced since he was 7, but his dad lived in town and he saw him a lot. He could talk to his dad about a lot of things, but he never had really talked to him much about sex. His dad had told him to use a condom, if he ever had sex, but that was about the whole sex talk. Brad broke down crying on the phone with his dad. His dad agreed to come and get him and take him to the doctor. And his dad agreed to talk to his mom for him.

The doctor confirmed that Brad had genital warts, and he had a couple more warts, too, near his anus. Brad was shattered. He felt crushed. He felt like he had only had sex one time, with one girl, and he would never be able to have sex again, because he didn't ever want to give warts to anyone nor did he ever feel like he could tell a girl he had it. Brad had bumps not just on his penis, but on his butt, where a condom would not cover it. All he could think about was that he felt he could never have sex again, with anyone, ever! His sex life was over and he was only 16! He could never, ever, take a chance of giving what he had to someone else—a sexually transmitted infection that lasts for life!

Brad had to make a second doctor's appointment to get the warts *burned off!* He had to go to a specialist, he had to have a shot right into his penis and another one near his anus, and then he had to have the warts burned off the tip of his penis! The whole appointment was horribly embarrassing and horribly painful, despite the medication. The top of his penis was literally scraped with a knife to remove the warts!

His dad made him call Tara and tell her about his genital warts diagnosis and outbreak. Brad was terrified. He felt like he was a big fool for getting warts, but since he was a virgin, he knew it wasn't from him! So, he called Tara. Tara started to cry. She wouldn't speak. Brad didn't know what to do, so he went over to her parent's house to talk to her. She was up in her room and wouldn't come downstairs. Finally, Tara's sister just let Brad in and he went to talk to her. It all came out that Tara knew she had warts: her boyfriend had given it to her, which he got when he cheated on her. It was the reason they broke up. Tara thought her "outbreak" was over and that Brad couldn't get it. Tara had never told Brad that she had it. She was very ashamed and didn't want to admit that she didn't tell him, but she told Brad she thought she was "safe" and that he wouldn't get it and that she could avoid telling him. Brad was outraged. He really wanted to hurt someone. He wanted to hurt Tara and he wanted to go beat up her ex-boyfriend, too. He was so mad, he couldn't speak to Tara anymore, and he left.

Brad's mom and dad found out that Tara gave him the STD and that she didn't even tell him when she knew she had it. They started talking about suing her or bringing a lawsuit against her. That talk died down after a few days, but everyone in the family was mad at Tara.

Actually, after a few days, Brad was mad with himself. He didn't do the one thing his dad had told him to do: wear a condom, although he wasn't sure that would have helped. Now, his sex life, he felt was ruined, and it had hardly started.

STDs, Safer Sex, and Birth Control

One of the worst things about having an STD is that you have to tell your future sexual partners that you have it. For Brad, the thought of having to tell someone he had warts was unbearable. The thought of not telling someone else was unthinkable. Embarrassed and unsure of what to do, Brad stayed away from relationships and from sex for a long time. Physically recovering from having the warts removed took a few weeks, and it was painful alone.

Condoms can help to prevent STDs, the spread of warts, but sometimes condoms don't cover the place where the blister or bump occurs on the pelvic area, vulva, or mouth. Although you can never have safe sex with someone who has warts, you can have safer sex, use a condom and never have sex during outbreaks.

HPV is becoming the most common sexually transmitted disease. Some girls and many guys are carriers of the disease, they don't have any symptoms and they don't even know they have it! The symptoms may not appear for weeks or months until one's immune system becomes distressed.

It is estimated as many as 50% of college-aged girls have HPV!

Think about it: if you have sexual intercourse with a college-aged girl, there is a high chance that she is infected with HPV, and she probably doesn't know that she has it! Without her even knowing it, she can give you HPV. In turn, any future sexual partner you have can get HPV, too.

Genital warts are caused by a virus called human papilloma virus, or HPV. HPV stays in a person's system for life, too, so warts can recur. While there are many different types of warts, genital warts can form and grow on a person's genitals, including the pelvic area, the anus, the vulva, and inside of the vagina. Genital warts are also very contagious and spread through skin-to-skin contact. Like herpes, they can be spread with oral-genital contact. Genital warts can be big or very small cauliflower-like bumps, that may form in clusters or a bunch all together. The bumps are usually painless, but they can itch. The warts have to be removed by a doctor, usually by being burned off, each and every one of them, which is very painful, due to the sensitivity in the region.

As with herpes, condoms can be used to give protection against genital warts, but the condom may give only partial protection. One of the bad things about HPV is that it has been associated with an increased risk of cervical cancer later in life for women. It has also been associated with cancer of the vulva, and anal cancer. For women, once they have been infected with warts, it is very important to have regular pelvic exams to check for problems throughout their life (Bell, 1998). Fortunately, a new vaccine for HPV, to help prevent getting the virus, will be available for girls soon.

Gonorrhea

Gonorrhea is another bacterial infection that is passed through penis-vagina intercourse, anal sex, and oral sex. Gonorrhea of the throat is becoming more common with the increase of oral sex, including more guys giving girls oral sex, and not realizing that STDs are spread from the transmission of bodily fluids, including in the mouth.

Oral sex is not safe sex!

Symptoms of gonorrhea, also known as "the clap" or "drip," include a funky smelling discharge with pus in it, and painful, burning urination. Many guys do not know they have it, and have no symptoms, and some girls have no symptoms, either. As with chlamydia, serious pelvic infections and scarring of the reproductive organs can

STDs, Safer Sex, and Birth Control

occur, causing infertility or an inability to have children. Gonorrhea can be treated with antibiotics, with both partners taking the drugs to get rid of it.

Hepatitis B

Hepatitis B is a virus that can infect a person's liver, causing a serious illness, and even death. Hepatitis B is spread through sexual practices that exchange bodily fluids, including kissing, all types of intercourse, oral sex, and sharing of blood. Hepatitis is common among intravenous drug users (injecting drugs into veins with a needle), and people who practice anal sex. Most people don't realize they have hepatitis because it is a lot like having the flu. Symptoms include a sick stomach, no appetite, headaches, dizziness, being tired, soreness in your liver area, dark-colored urine, and yellowish eyes or skin. Hepatitis B is usually curable, but the medical treatment is very long and extensive, including two to three months of treatment (Bell, 1998).

> It is highly recommended that young adults get vaccinated against Hepatitis B, as it is an easy way to prevent a disease that can have many complications and kill you.

Pubic Lice

Commonly known as "crabs," these are tiny little animals that jump from one body to another, and generally live in hair, including pubic hair and eyelashes. Pubic lice are highly contagious and spread from close contact with another person who has them. You will know if you have crabs because they itch like crazy! This condition is treatable and curable, with over-the-counter and prescription drugs. You can ask your pharmacist for help or go to a doctor. It is really important that all of your clothing, bedding, carpeting, stuffed animals, or anything cloth be cleaned in hot soapy water or put in tightly sealed plastic bags to totally get rid of all the little bugs and their eggs, which can live for days.

Syphilis

Another bacterial infection, syphilis is spread by sexual or skin contact from a person who has the rash or sores of the disease. Drugs can completely cure the illness, if it is caught in an early stage. Untreated, syphilis is a very serious, life-threatening disease, causing damage to internal organs, including your sexual organs, and causing birth defects. Later, it can also damage the heart, brain, and nervous system, even leading to insanity. Early treatment is very important.

SAFEST SEX

There is no such thing as totally safe sex with a partner.

If you are engaging in sexual practices, you are taking a risk that you will get an STD or get a girl pregnant.

Abstinence. The absolute surest way to avoid ever contracting an STD or having an unwanted pregnancy is to not be sexually active, which is called sexual abstinence, or literally, abstaining from sex. The safest sexual activity is to participate in sexual behaviors that do not allow the transmission of fluids between two partners. Also, do not kiss anyone who has a cold sore or fever blister. The safest sex is where you do not engage in any skin to skin contact of the genitals, including not kissing or touching the genitals with the mouth. For example, sexual contact with each other's genitals through clothing, by touching or rubbing each other through clothing, is a safe way to express sexual affection. Dry kissing (no tongue), holding, or dancing, as long as sexual fluids are not exchanged and sexual skin does not touch, are safe sexual behaviors.

Some people are afraid of getting AIDS from wet kissing, but most doctors believe the quality of the HIV virus in saliva is too low to cause HIV. Abstinence is effective as safest sex only if it is practiced *each* and *every* time. Period. It is important to know that many teenagers plan to abstain from sex, and to be safe from sexual risks through sexual abstinence, but for a thousand different reasons, this plan changes. Abstinence is only effective if is it used continuously, or all the time, which, in reality, often does not happen. For that reason, it is important to have a back-up plan, in case you change your mind in a given situation.

Masturbation: Having sex with yourself poses no threat of acquiring a sexually transmitted disease. Masturbation in front of your partner, without touching each other or sharing sexual fluids, is also safe sex.

SAFER SEX PRACTICES

You can be responsible for yourself and you can learn to practice "safer" sex. You can learn what is sexually dangerous or risky and *not* engage in those behaviors. Sometimes people practice safe sex or safer sex almost all the time, but then they have a bad day, or get drunk, or have a great day and a moment of passion and all thoughts of safe sex go out the window. Sometimes it is just a matter of a moment, or sometimes you're just angry and tell yourself, "Oh, what the hell, I'll take the chance," and just do whatever you think you want to do without thinking about the consequences.

In the movies, in a moment of passion, the couple rarely stops when they're slammed up against the wall or falling on a bed and says, "Hey, we've got to get some protection first." Or, "Look, you don't have any STDs or anything, do you?" In real life, you can and should stop and ask. A lot of guys are too embarrassed to stop and ask a girl to put on a condom, and a lot of girls are too afraid to ask, too. In truth, girls will be very relieved that you asked, that you did something to help protect both of you, and no, it won't ruin the whole thing.

Safer Sex Guide

- Start with sexual relations negotiations. Discuss with your partner: STDs, safer sex and sexual practices, the use of condoms, cheating (sex with others outside of the relationship), and birth control.

- Practice monogamy. Monogamy means two people only have sex with each other. If both of you are absolutely certain neither of you is infected with an STD, and you are certain neither of you has any other partners (which can be very hard to know because of the honesty issue, even when you love each other), then you will both be safer from STDs.

- Use a condom each and every time there is sexual contact of the genitals, including oral and anal sex.

- Identify your own past potentially risky sexual behaviors. If there is any risk, see a doctor or visit a clinic before having unprotected sex.

- Don't wait, don't worry, get tested, first, before you have sex again!

- Ask your sexual partners about their potential risk of disease. If there is any risk, have your partner visit a clinic or see a doctor for STD testing before you consent to have sex with them.

STDs, Safer Sex, and Birth Control

- Limit your sexual partners. The more sexual partners you have, the greater your chance for STDs.

- Also for this reason, avoid partners who have had multiple partners.

- Postpone any exchange of bodily fluids until lab tests verify that you are both free of STDs. HIV testing, for example, is a two-step process, and you have to wait six months for your second HIV test to be reasonably certain that you do not have the virus.

- At first, try taking a bath or shower together and examine each other's genitals. Make sure your partner's genitals are free of bumps, raw redness, or sores. Many STDs cannot be seen upon examination, but some, such as genital warts or some herpes sores, can be seen.

- Wear condoms whenever you have penis-vagina, penis-anus, penis-mouth, or vagina-vagina sex. Anal sex is more risky.

- After sex, urinate and wash your genitals with warm soapy water to wash out bacterial organisms.

- Don't use IV (intravenous or "shooting up" with a needle) drugs.

- Don't share needles, whether injecting drugs or piercing your body for a tattoo. Make sure all equipment is cleaned and sterilized before using it.

- Don't think you are safe from AIDS if you don't use needles Do not share belongings that can have body fluids on them, like toothbrushes or razors.

- Avoid sex with people who have STDs, prostitutes, and IV drug users.

> Assume your sexual partner has an STD and take the appropriate precautions: use a condom or do not exchange body fluids.

BIRTH CONTROL AND PREGNANCY

Both girls and guys are responsible for planning for birth control and preventing STDs and pregnancy. Unfortunately, as was discussed in Chapter Three, no matter how educated and smart guys are, many of them are very interested in having sexual relations with girls, but they leave the birth control and STD prevention up to the girl. In fact, some guys take pride in saying, "I will never wear a condom." Many guys want sex, but won't take the responsibility of the potential consequences of sex, which includes the risk of pregnancy. Many guys expect girls to take care of the birth control, and then "take care of it" if they are pregnant.

While a pregnancy will not change a guy's life in the same way as it will change a girl's life, an unplanned pregnancy will most certainly affect your life. Chapter Four discussed the four options of an unplanned pregnancy, including what each of those options mean to a young man. This section will discuss how to best prevent an unplanned pregnancy, as well as some other factors that unwed fathers need to know. Every young man ought to think about the potential of pregnancy and the responsibility it could carry for him for many years.

A Guy's Guide to an Unplanned Pregnancy

So, what happens when your girlfriend gets pregnant? One in three girls gets pregnant by the time she is 20 years old. A very real chance exists that your girlfriend will be one of these girls. The four options for dealing with an unplanned pregnancy are reviewed below.

1. She has an abortion, which is totally *her* choice.
2. She has the baby, raises it herself: you pay child support.
3. She has the baby and she makes a plan for its adoption.
4. She has the baby and you get married or live together.

Guy's Reactions to Finding Out about Pregnancy

- **Shock.** Most guys are shocked when they find out their girl-friend, or a girl they had sex with, is pregnant, even though they shouldn't be.
- **Fear.** From mild to extreme concerns over what to do.
- **Denial.** "How do I know it's mine?" Questioning your paternity. Denial, when you *know* it's your baby, can be cruel and like rejection. However, it is important to make sure you are the father. Blood tests and DNA testing, in cases of uncertain paternity, can determine who is the father, both before and after a baby is born.
- **Pride and joy.** Sometimes young men are delighted with the pregnancy and take pride in their manhood, bragging that they are fathers.
- **Rejection of the girl.** "If you have the baby, I won't have anything to do with you."
- **Abandon the girl.** Running away and trying to pretend it isn't happening. Don't answer phone calls, stop seeing her, or even leave town.
- **Stay in denial.** Get drunk or high for days or weeks to forget about it.
- **Act supportive.** "What would *you* like to do?" Talking to the girl and/or her parents about options. Being emotionally supportive, even when you are afraid of what to do.
- **Fear of being trapped into marriage.** About 30% of young men marry their teenage, pregnant girlfriend.

Most of the time, even in the best case scenario, even when a guy knows he's the father of the child and even when he knows he loves the girls, most guys are very scared and don't know what to do. Fear drives all the bad reactions of denial, rejection, abandonment, going on drunken binges, and running away from the situation.

The best way a guy can handle an unwanted pregnancy is to face the truth, confirm the pregnancy, and stay close to the girl to make decisions about which of the four options above, is best for everyone, to handle the situation. When guys run away from the problem, the problem can get bigger in the long run. If a guy runs away and the girl has an abortion, he can feel a lot of guilt for abandoning her. Also, if the girl wants to choose abortion and doesn't have the money to pay for it, and the guy wants that too, he loses his chances of helping her get an abortion. If the girl doesn't have an abortion and she has your child, sooner or later the situation is going to catch up to you, even if you try to run from it. About one third of teen pregnancies end in abortion, but that rate varies greatly on the ethnicity of the mother. Many more pregnant white girls have abortions than black and Hispanic girls (www.guttmacher.org).

If abortion isn't the option chosen, you will become a father, and you will have the responsibility to support your child, unless plans are made for the child's adoption. One of the biggest responsibilities that scare young men is financial support, since you'll probably have to pay child support. Even with a child support court order, a guy might say, "I will never pay child support." However, it is amazing what a night in jail will do to change a father's mind. Of course, as discussed in Chapter Four, there are other responsibilities to being a father, caring for a child, and providing emotional support to the mother.

Also, if you become a father, even though at first, most guys reject the idea, somewhere later down the line you might change your mind and realize this baby is your child. You might want to be a part of this child's life, or might want to have a choice in whether or not the child is adopted. Fathers can lose their rights to being a father when the mother makes plans for a child's adoption, and terminates a father's rights to his child. Losing a child, even though you really didn't plan for or want that child, can also be emotionally devastating. Treating a mother poorly or cruelly when you find out about the pregnancy can turn the mother and child against you (and their family). If you run away in the beginning, you might lose your choices later, like with Carlos.

An Unwed Father—Carlos' Story

Carlos was 17 when he fathered a child. He had a sexual relationship with a girl from "the barrio," or what some people would call "the other side of the tracks," or the Hispanic ghetto. Carlos had a girlfriend, but they didn't have a sexual relationship. Carlos was Catholic and according to his faith, he and his girlfriend decided to wait until marriage to have sex. Carlos had a secret girlfriend with whom he had sex, and had unprotected sex.

Carlos' other girlfriend Theresa, or who he really just considered a girl he had sex with, was 15 when she got pregnant. Theresa told Carlos about missing her period and that she was afraid she was pregnant. At first, Carlos waited to see if she was really pregnant. When he found out she really was and that she was going to have the baby, he stayed away from her.

Carlos never told his girlfriend, nor his parents. He acted like it never happened and went on with his life, secretly fearing someone, especially his girlfriend, would find out. Months passed and no one found out. Theresa tried to call Carlos and even tried to see him once, showing up at his school, but Carlos told her to leave him alone, he denied that it was his baby, and he told Theresa to go away.

When Theresa had her baby, she called Carlos. Carlos refused to even go to the hospital to see his baby daughter. Finally, Theresa's mother called Carlos' mother and told her what had happened. Carlo's mother was shocked and angry and ashamed of what Carlos had done. She went to go to see her granddaughter in the hospital, and she made Carlos go with her.

By the time they got to the hospital, they found out that Theresa had made plans to give the baby up for adoption. Theresa's mother was very poor, and she was too sick to work and was on disability and her father was dead. They had no family in the United States and no money to return to their family. While she was pregnant, Theresa had turned to an adoption agency to help pay for her care, including getting money to pay for their rent, her clothes, food, and medical expenses. In return, she was planning to give up her baby for adoption.

Carlos' family was extremely upset. Adoption was not an option for their family. Adoption was unheard of and they would not agree with it. Carlos' family encouraged him to not sign the papers, not sign away his parental rights, and they would agree to take care of the baby.

Unfortunately, in their state, if the father does not acknowledge paternity (that he is the father), does not help the mother at all during pregnancy, by helping with food, clothes, care, does not visit the mother, or at least, even as a teenager, try to help the pregnant mother, the state can file a petition to terminate a father's parental rights, without even notifying him! Carlo's name was put on a notification of adoption list and didn't register as the baby's father, since he was not acknowledging he was the father during the entire pregnancy. Theresa tried to tell him, but he refused to return her phone calls. Once that was done, Carlo's parental rights could be terminated, without his actually signing away his parental rights.

That is exactly what happened! Theresa and Carlos' baby was adopted and there was nothing Carlos could do about it after the baby was born. Carlos' family tried to hire an attorney to stop the adoption, but, in their state, it was too late! Carlos had no rights as an "unwed father."

Carlos' family was devastated. They felt a great loss that a child of their family would be adopted, out in the world, and they could do nothing about it. Even Carlos, after he saw his daughter, had deep regrets about what he did. Plus, Carlos' girlfriend found out all about it and she broke off their relationship. Carlos loved his girlfriend and had since childhood: he was devastated over losing her and she would not forgive him or take him back. Months and a few years later, Carlos regretted abandoning Theresa, and ultimately losing his daughter.

Carlo's advice to other teens: Don't run away from a girl, who is pregnant with your child. You don't know how you will feel when the baby is born. You might change your mind. Your family may want to help you. Don't make the same mistake I made. I didn't know I couldn't change the past.

WHAT EVERY GUY NEEDS TO KNOW ABOUT GIRLS AND BIRTH CONTROL

By now, it should seem very clear to you that, as a young man, it is your job to take responsibility for your own sexual behavior, and plan to preventing pregnancy or choose to abstain from sexual activity, at least until you are ready to take that responsibility very seriously. The only birth control methods a man really has control over are abstinence, condoms, withdrawal, spermicide, and later in life, sterilization (having a vasectomy). All of the birth control methods will be discussed in this chapter, but as a guy, you need to know what you can control, to control your future.

> The best way to avoid an unplanned pregnancy, is
> to choose abstinence, or to plan for birth control. If
> you don't plan it, don't plan to prevent pregnancy.

Trusting Girls with Birth Control

Every guy should be very cautious to not trust that a girl will take care of birth control, even if she says she will. Although this sounds negative toward girls, as a teenage guy, it is unwise and probably stupid to totally trust a teenage girl (or even a grown woman who wants a baby) about birth control, especially if don't know her very, very well. Even if your girlfriend is very responsible with birth control, or is taking birth control shots (see Depo shots below), or she is using one of the methods below, as a guy, if you want to be as sure as possible that she will not get pregnant, you should not completely leave birth control up to her. An unplanned pregnancy, as you know, affects your future: take charge of your future, by playing it very safe. You can always use more than one birth control method at one time: if you use a condom and the pill together, you will be 99.9% protected from pregnancies and from STDs at the same time!

Teenage girls can be unpredictable. They can change their minds easily, they can lose their tempers easily, they can make more mistakes than adult women, and to be honest, more than a few girls can be manipulative and vindictive. Until you can totally trust a girl, which can take a very long relationship to develop that trust, like a year or more, trust yourself, while you are developing your trust with her, too.

Top Reasons to Not Trust Girls with Birth Control

Girls Who Trap Guys into Fatherhood

- Some girls want to get pregnant. As unbelievable as this might be, some girls want to be mothers and they don't care if they get pregnant or not. Girls that don't have other goals and plans in their life, like going to college or finishing high school or getting a career, may think that motherhood sounds like a good idea.
- Watch out for girls whose friends already have children. They might want to have a child because that is what their friends are doing and they want to have a child, too.
- Some girls want to get a guy by having his child. Some girls think that if they get pregnant, it is a way to hold on to a guy, to have a long term relationship, to always have that guy in their life, or to force him into marrying her.
- Some girls don't realize that trapping a guy into marriage, in reality, traps them into parenthood. They might not think that far into the future about the realities about parenting.
- Some girls glamorize motherhood and parenthood, not realizing what it takes to take care of a child. In some cases, when a girl doesn't feel loved or a sense of belonging with her family, she might want to have a baby to "have someone who loves her."
- Some girls with bad home lives may see pregnancy as a way out of the house, by having you support them.
- Some girls see having a child as a way to get a child support check, which might be another way to have money to support themselves, to give them an income or increase their income.

Girls Who Are Irresponsible About Taking or Using Birth Control

- Some girls simply do not understand how birth control really works and they might make a mistake. For example, one girl thought she just took the Pill on the days she had sex, not every day.

- Some girls are very forgetful and irresponsible about taking daily medication.
- Some girls don't have the money or are not organized enough to get their birth control and it runs out or they just didn't get around to getting it.
- Some girls will not consistently use certain types of birth control, like a diaphragm.

Birth Control Failure/Other

- Used improperly or inconsistently, birth control can have higher failure rates than those stated by birth control types.
- Some girls simply are very fertile and are more likely to get pregnant, despite the proper use of birth control.
- Medications, like antibiotics can affect the failure rate of birth control, and many people don't know about these "other drug effects."
- Every birth control method has a failure rate. Read below to learn about "effective" and "failure" rates.
- Some girls will lie and say they are pregnant to get a guy to "pay for abortion," when they aren't pregnant, to get money from them.

> It is a very good idea to make sure you trust a girl in other ways, beside with birth control, before you trust her with your future.

How To Know If You Can Trust a Girl

- She makes promises and keeps them
- She doesn't lie
- She doesn't manipulate you in other ways, like play mind games
- She is not a drama queen (at least not very often)

- She has a good reputation with her friends
- Your friends like her and trust her (listen to your friends)
- She doesn't have a past with guys where they all hate her
- She has never cheated on you
- She doesn't push you away from your friends (too much)
- You feel comfortable with her
- She is your best friend

Methods of Birth Control

This section includes all the different types of birth control available to men, but mostly women to prevent pregnancy. This section describes different types of birth control, and also tells approximately how effective each type is when used. Effectiveness is how well birth control will protect you against pregnancy. The effectiveness of a birth control method is an approximation, or an estimate, based on how well it works for many women, depending on how well the birth control method is actually used.

There are two different rates of effectiveness for birth control: "typical use" and "perfect use." Typical use means how the birth control method is usually used by real people in real situations. Perfect use is the effectiveness of a birth control method when it is used *each and every time in the correct way*, exactly how it is supposed to be used. For each birth control method, a statistic will be given for how many women get pregnant each year for every 100 women using that method of birth control (Planned Parenthood, 1999). For example, with male condoms, when they are used "perfectly," they are 97% effective. This means that 3% or 3 women in 100 will become pregnant each year. However, with "typical use" condoms are 86% effective, meaning 14 out of 100 women will get pregnant each year, using this birth control method. As you can see, how well a birth control device is used makes a huge difference on whether or not it will work! Birth control has to be used right, and used each and every time.

Some types of birth control are available at any local drugstore or the local health department. Some types of birth control require a doctor's prescription. To get a doctor's prescription, a girl has to go to a doctor's and get a special type of physical exam, called a "gynecological exam." Ideally, a girl will get her first gynecological exam before she becomes sexually active. In a gynecological exam, a doctor will examine a girl's genitals and make sure everything is healthy and working right, as well as discuss birth control options, before she is sexually active. After a girl is first sexually active, she should definitely start having a gynecological exam once a year.

No Method of Birth Control

When no method of birth control is used, up to 90% of sexually active girls will become pregnant in one year. This means that in any given year, 90 out of 100 girls who do not use any type of birth control will become pregnant.

Abstinence

Abstinence is simply not having sexual intercourse ever, under any circumstances. Pregnancy can't happen if sperm is kept out of a girl's vagina. My dad's entire sex talk to me when I was a teenager was, "Abstinence is the only 100% way to prevent pregnancy." He was right. Looking around at my 8 brothers and sisters, for whom we had nicknames, "Miss Pill," "Miss IUD," and "Mr. Diaphagm," noted for birth control failures: I believed him.

Perfect use of abstinence for birth control has a 0% pregnancy rate, but abstinence must be used each and every time to be effective. "Periodic abstinence" is more commonly or typically used for birth control. Periodic abstinence means that even though people vow that they will not have sex, the vow of abstinence, such as the vow of abstinence from smoking or drinking or speeding, is typically broken with alarming frequency. When one doesn't expect to have sex and uses this as the only birth control method, with no backup method, the failure rate is 20%. Using periodic abstinence as their only means of birth control, 20 percent of girls will become pregnant in one year.

Outercourse

Outercourse is sexual play that does not involve penis-vagina or anal intercourse. Sex play may include vaginal, oral, or anal sexual stimulation. For most people, this means kissing, hugging, touching, sexual touching or rubbing with hands, oral sex, "dry humping," and mutual masturbation. Outercourse is nearly 100% effective in preventing pregnancy. Caution: Pregnancy is still possible if semen or "pre-ejaculate," contacts the vulva. Pre-ejaculate is a small amount of semen that is discharged from the penis (that tiny drop of fluid on the tip of your penis), that a guy gets when he is sexually excited but hasn't yet ejaculated or come.

Outercourse is effective against HIV and STDs as well as long as bodily fluids are NOT exchanged through oral or anal sex or by skin-to-skin contact through small, even microscopic, cuts or openings of the skins, such as blisters or sores.

The Pill

The birth control pill is the most popular method of birth control for teenagers. As stated above, a gynecological exam and a prescription for pills is required. Some health insurance plans pay for birth control pills, and some teen clinics give them away for free. The pill is a hormone used to prevent ovulation, so that pregnancy is not possible. It prevents the egg from being released from the ovaries, so there is no egg to fertilize and impregnate with sperm. It is a highly effective method of birth control, when used consistently and correctly.

Some girls have side effects from hormones and can't take the pill, so they need to talk to their health care professional about this. The birth control patch and ring work in similar hormonal ways as the pill, although they put the hormones in your body differently. Talk to your health care professional to see if these options are right for your sexual partner. With perfect use, the pill is 99.5% effective. Typical use has 95% effectiveness.

Condoms

Condoms are available over the counter at drug stores, some super-markets, women's clinics, the local health clinic, and even Wal-Mart. The condom is called a "barrier" method of birth control, meaning there is a barrier preventing sperm from fertilizing the egg and causing pregnancy. A condom is a sheath, like a fitted balloon that covers the penis, made of latex, plastic, or animal tis-sue. Condoms, when used consistently, can be highly effective in preventing pregnancy and protecting against STDs. Female con-doms are shaped to fit inside a woman's vagina and protect against pregnancy and STDs in the same manner, by providing a barrier to keep sperm from fertilizing the egg. Female condoms can be used for heterosexual or homosexual sexual activities. Male condoms with perfect use have 97% effectiveness: however, typical use ef-fectiveness is 86%.

Diaphragm and Cervical Cap

Both of these birth control devices are obtained by prescription, from a doctor or nurse practitioner, following a gynecological exam, for women to use. It is a "barrier" method made of latex, and it is specifically fitted to your size. These devices are inserted into a girl's vagina and fit over her cervix. The cervical opening leads to the uterus, where an egg can be fertilized to cause pregnancy. The barrier blocks semen from entering your uterus. These methods also use a spermicidal jelly to kill sperm, so it can't fertilize an egg.

A diaphragm or cervical cap can be used over and over again. These devices are fitted for a woman by a doctor so that they will fit the woman's individual cervix size (and there are many different sizes). Most pregnancies occur with these devices because a woman either doesn't use it or she doesn't know a spermicidal jelly has to be used with it every time in order for it to be effective. Most commonly, in the passion of the sexual moment, one of these devices is simply not used. A diaphragm or cervical cap must be used *each and every time* sexual intercourse occurs to be effective. Perfect use is 96% effective for a diaphragm, and 94% effective for a cervical cap. Typical use is 81% effective for a diaphragm and 80% effective for a cervical cap. As you can see, these methods can be highly effective when used all the time and correctly, but they have a significantly high failure rate, or cases of pregnancy, when they are not used all the time. Using a diaphragm or cervical cap, in combination with a condom is a good idea for a very high rate of birth control effectiveness.

Intrauterine Device or IUD

An IUD, or intrauterine device, must be obtained by prescription from a doctor or nurse practitioner, and the prescription is followed by gynecological exam. An IUD is a small plastic device fitted and placed inside a woman's uterus. It can be left in place five to ten years, but it needs to be checked at least every two years. An IUD is the world's most frequently used reversible method of birth control. It works by not allowing the egg to implant on the uterine wall. It is not intended for teenagers to use—it is generally recommended for women in monogamous relationships who already have children, as some women can in rare situations develop infections and sterility. Perfect and typical uses of an IUD device are both close to 99% effectiveness.

Contraceptive Foams, Gels, and Suppositories

Contraceptive foams, gels, and suppositories are available without a doctor's prescription from a drug store or grocery store. All of these methods work as spermicides, which means they kill sperm. When used alone, these methods are about as effective as condoms. *Used with condoms, they are 99% effective—nearly as effective as the pill!* The use of condoms and spermicides, when used together and used each and every time, are highly effective in preventing pregnancy, and you can easily get these at your local grocery or drug store, without having to go to a doctor or get a prescription, making this method of birth control easily accessible for young men. Some people may have an allergic reaction or irritation from latex or certain types of spermicides. Changing your brand may solve the problem. On the lighter side, one girl shared a funny story about contraceptive foam, saying it worked fine, but it made noises during sex because of the "foaminess" with the vaginal lubrication, making sounds during intercourse like a churning washing machine.

Norplant

Norplant used to be obtained from a doctor or nurse following a gynecological exam. A six-capsule hormonal implant was inserted under the skin of the upper arm. Like the pill, this method of birth control was reversible, but it had to be removed from under your skin. It was removed from the U.S. market in 2002. However, as its effects last for five years, some implants may be in circulation still.

Depo-Provera

Depo-Provera is an injectable hormone that lasts 12 weeks. The girl has to get an exam and see a doctor or nurse, who will give her a shot in her arm. This method is a very effective and convenient method of birth control. It affects her body like the pill, preventing ovulation (eggs being released from the ovaries), so she can't get pregnant.

The advantage to Depo-Provera shots is that the girl doesn't have to remember to take a pill every day. She will have to go to the doctor or clinic once every three months. As a guy, if your partner wants to use "Depo" shots for birth control, you can go to the clinic with her, watch her get her shot, and be sure she is really on birth control, without worrying about whether or not she is taking her pills correctly. Plus, girls often like it when their boyfriend will accompany them to the doctor and participate in obtaining birth control.

There may be side effects, however, as with all birth control pills. Another negative aspect of Depo shots is that there is no way to stop the possible side effects until the shot wears off in 12 to 14 weeks. For some girls, it is a good idea to try birth control pills first to see if they have any negative side effects, before trying shots. Also, it is very important to make sure the Depo shot is given very regularly or a lapse of time can result in pregnancy.

Withdrawal

Withdrawal is also known as "pulling out." Pulling out or withdrawing means a guy removes his penis from the girl's vagina just prior to ejaculating his semen when he has an orgasm. Used perfectly, withdrawal has an effectiveness rate of 96%. Typical use of withdrawal has an 81% effectiveness rate. This means that, every year, 19 out of 100 girls counting on withdrawal will get pregnant. Withdrawal is a very risky method of birth control for young people. Mostly, this is because young men often have poor control over their ability to control their ejaculation. Basically, many young men do not know exactly when they are going to come or how fast they will come, and predicting the moment to pull out can be very tricky and unreliable. Also, some foolish, often drunk guys will think, "Oh, who cares, I'm going to go for it," and decide to come inside the girl. Also, a girl can get pregnant from "pre-ejaculate," (which is explained above, under outercourse), since the pre-ejaculate is present every time withdrawal is used. The withdrawal method is better than using no method of birth control at all, but it is a very risky method of birth control for preventing pregnancy for young women.

Emergency Contraception

This is commonly called "the morning-after pill." This is an available method for women if contraception fails, like if a condom breaks, if the guy didn't pull out, you didn't use the diaphragm in a moment of passion, or if any type of unexpected, unprotected sex takes place. It is very effective if taken within 72 hours of unprotected sex. Sometimes, a woman has to go to a health clinic or doctor's office to receive this treatment. In some states, it is available directly from a pharmacy without a prescription, just by asking the pharmacist for the medication. Even in states where it is legal to obtain emergency contraception from a pharmacy, some pharmacies, due to their ethical beliefs, that using it is similar to have a very early abortion, will not carry it. If one doesn't have it, try another pharmacy, or call around to find a pharmacy who does keep it in stock.

Sterilization

Sterilization is the most widely used form of birth control, but it is almost always reserved for men and women who are much older, and it is almost always inappropriate for teenagers. Sterilization is a permanent surgical procedure to prevent pregnancy, and it is frequently irreversible. You shouldn't even think about getting sterilized or agree that your partner undergo sterilization until you are absolutely certain that you do not want any more children; most doctors will not perform this surgery until you have had children and/or you are well over 30 years old. Sterilization may be possible to reverse in some cases, but the procedure is very expensive and reversals only work 25% of the time. "Vasectomy" is the term for a man's sterilization procedure. This is where the tubes that carry sperm for ejaculation are permanently cut and blocked. "Tubal ligation" is the term for women's sterilization. This is where the tubes that carry eggs, the fallopian tubes, are cut and blocked.

Natural Family Planning

Also called "fertility awareness methods," these methods do not involve pills or devices. Natural family planning includes several different methods, which are most effective when used together. These methods are called: post-ovulation, cervical mucous or ovulation, calendar or rhythm, and thermal or basal body temperature. A fertile woman's body gives off subtle signs of fertility during the menstrual cycle which can be tracked to determine when a woman will get pregnant. These methods have a relatively high failure rate, and require a great deal of responsibility to be used correctly. It is highly recommended that if you choose these methods, you obtain detailed instruction and information from a health care educator concerning proper use. Since teenagers often have irregular periods, it is recommended that you consider other methods of birth control. Typical use of natural family planning methods have 90 to 99% effectiveness rates.

EIGHT

PURE VIRGIN SEX: SEX FOR THE FIRST TIME AND BEYOND

221

The truth is: Millions of girls and guys get hurt by sex. Engaging in sexual intercourse, with no guidance nor past sexual experiences is like trying to drive on a major highway during rush hour when you have never driven behind the wheel of a car. One would expect a lot of mistakes, wrong turns and painful accidents.

Guys are physically driven to sex. Guys are pulled along, like the current of the ocean at high tide, both physically and emotionally toward sex. The wonderful difference between guys and sharks in the sea, is that young men have minds that can change the tide of emotions and hormones, think about how to use and enjoy this fantastic sexual drive, and make it a joyful part of life, for themselves and their partners, for the first time and beyond.

Pure virgin sex is all about giving guys guidance to know how to have a healthy sexual beginning, for themselves, and for their partners, so neither of them get hurt by sex. A lot of teenagers and adults have relationship and sexual problems, but the truth is that many of these problems can be avoided!

As teenagers, guys usually get hurt by making sexual mistakes (see Chapter Four on the Top Ten Sexual Mistakes Guys Make), getting hurt emotionally, or by hurting a girl, both emotionally or physically. When guys hurt girls, in the long run, they can get hurt by a girl that got hurt by a guy that got hurt by a girl that got hurt by a guy, and so on and so on.

Most guys do not want to hurt girls. Most guys are really sweet, wonderful, good guys who like girls but they are also guys who are driven by male hormones, think about sex a lot, who are wired to want sex, and who often think they want to have sex as soon as the first opportunity arises. First, guys need to make sure they know how to treat a girl right (see Chapter Two). Next, guys need to know if they're ready for sex (see Chapter Four). Then, if one at least believes they are ready for sex and ready to have a relationship with a girl, a guy needs to know physically how have a sexual relationship with a girl, when she is ready, so both can experience sexuality in a positive, healthy way.

> If everyone starts out their sexual lives experiencing sex positively, an amazing and important change will happen in our world: More people will enjoy sex and have opportunities for indescribably incredible relationships in life!

Everywhere you look: on T.V., MTV, the Internet, magazines, books, and in every day conversation, people are talking about and writing about sex, mostly on how to get more of it and do it better. If you have the right start, from the start, you won't need to figure out how to fix up your mess ups—so begin by knowing what you're doing before you do it. Sadly, many girls and guys are hurt by sex by not knowing what they are doing! Physically, a girl can get hurt by sex when a guy is sexually inexperienced or misinformed about how to have sex, especially sex for the first time. Emotionally, girls can get fears about sex that last for many years. One of the big reasons women seem to play games with sex or hate sex, especially later in life, is because when they had first sexual experiences, they learned to be turned off by sex.

> One of the greatest gifts in life can be destroyed because of the mistakes teens make when they are first having sexual experiences.

Since the majority of teens (80%) have their first sexual experiences as teenagers, including sexual intercourse, *Virgin Sex* provides information for teens and young adults to use whenever they first choose to experience sex, or lose their virginity, when they need this information the most. This chapter, in particular, provides real sex ed that may be difficult or impossible to receive at home or at school, about having sex for the first time and beyond. The overall goal is to empower you with knowledge that will help you have essential detailed sexual information, that even many adults don't have, to understand sex, from both an emotional and physical side, and guide you to have pure virgin sex and beyond.

PART I: THE EMOTIONAL SIDE OF SEX

Your experience with sex will depend on your emotions, not just on the physical side of sex. Her experience will depend on her emotions, too. How you feel about yourself, your partner, your situation, and your values, on any given day, with any given person, in any situation will depend on how you both feel, much more so than what you think you know about sex or certain sexual moves.

Most of the guys who tell their stories in this book, have told you to wait to have sex with someone you love. Like John, in Chapter

One said, "Wait until you find someone you really care about and that makes all the difference!" Buy why? Why do emotions make so much difference? It's all the same sexual wiring regardless of who is turning it on, right? Why would sex feel any different, depending on who you're having sex with? Sex is sex, right? For some guys, maybe, but for most guys, no, when they experience sex with deeper emotions attached.

Having feelings for someone changes sex into something different: Something better.

As you get older, it is likely that you will experience deeper, more complex and intense feelings toward someone else, although, some teenagers can have very real, very deep emotional and sexual attractions, too. Most guys will admit that waiting to have sex with someone they love or sincerely care about, is worth the wait. Even for guys who didn't wait until they were in love, when they had sex for the first time with someone just for the sexual experience, they later realize that sex with love, is better, and often regret not waiting.

Jealousy

Sex can make you feel good, but it can also make you feel very bad. Sex changes the way some people feel toward each other, especially for girls, but also for guys. Sex can make you feel all mixed up about people, relationships, and life.

For guys, once they are involved sexually, some experience one very new emotion: Jealousy.

As soon as a guy has sex with a girl, especially someone he has real affection and loving feelings toward, his feelings can change. As a teenager, your emotions can go a little wild and you might find yourself acting a tiny bit crazy. You might feel jealous. For some guys, after jealousy, comes possessiveness. Young guys often start acting as if they want to control a girl: what she wears (nothing too sexy or revealing), who she talks to, wanting to check her cell phone call list, reading her text messages, wondering where she's been, or asking when she's getting home. Really, guys don't know how to handle this new emotion of jealousy. Some guys can even get physically violent, when they never were before, like punch a hole in the wall when a girl treats them badly or even talks to another guy. Most guys are not prepared for feeling this strongly about anything in their life. Suddenly the "whatever," attitude you once had toward life or toward girls, turns into intense feelings. Jealousy is the kind of emotional change sex can have on a guy. That is why a lot of people say you should wait to have sex until you are "emotionally ready" for sex.

Emotional Trust: The "C" Word

Honestly, a lot of guys think they are ready for sex when a girl says, "Yes!" However, sex is a lot better for guys when they truly have feelings for a girl and you can trust her (see Chapter Seven, on how to know if you can trust a girl). The biggest clue to knowing if you are ready emotionally to be with someone sexually is whether or not you feel "comfortable," with a girl.

> The "L" word, love, is hard to define, even for adults, but the "C" word means feeling comfortable: when you can say anything you want and you can be yourself.

It's easy to know when you simply feel comfortable with a girl, as well as really liking her or loving her or even feeling like you're ready for sex. If you trust a girl, and you both care for each other, and you're comfortable with saying how you feel with her, it is much more likely that she will be considerate and caring of your feelings when it comes to sex, including normal jealousy. A girl is not as likely to be a big time flirt in front of your best friend, if she knows that bothers you, if you were comfortable enough to tell her how you feel. This is where having loving feelings toward each other truly makes sharing your sexuality emotionally safe and special. When you are comfortable talking about your feelings, and being yourself, you can both have the emotional trust you need for sex.

Girls and the Emotional-Sexual Connection

> For most girls, they want an emotional connection first, then maybe a sexual one. For most guys, they want a sexual connection first, then maybe an emotional one.

While this is a general statement about all guys and girls, generally it is true. Whether you are 15 or 55, it is very important to remember: if you want to have a sexual relationship with a woman, she will want and need to have an emotional relationship and connection, before she will think about having a sexual relationship with you. If you ever want or expect to have a sexual relationship or even any sexual encounter on any given day, most girls want to feel that emotional connection first. Even if you've had a sexual relationship for a long time, most girls need to have an emotional connection, before they will even have a sexual thought or feeling on that day or in that moment.

Some guys simply don't think about girls and their feelings. Their biological drive tells them that they want to have sex, period. However, you need to wait until the girl is ready, emotionally, for sex. Some guys (and men!) get pretty frustrated that they have to "go through hoops," usually meaning emotional hoops, to have a sexual relationship.

> Most girls need to be in the right emotional mood to want to have sex. Girls need to feel loved and to feel ongoing physical affection, not just affection that leads to sex.

Girls need to feel that emotional and physical connection of affection to feel sexual desire. Learning to show affection in little ways will lead to more emotional closeness and desire for you physically, later, if it's going to happen. It is very important to show physical affection, such as hugging, kissing, and touching with affection that doesn't lead right to sex. Girls also need to be treated right, so that they are not mad at you, which is a sexual turn-off. Anger is not a sexual turn-off for guys, but it definitely is for girls. If you are in a fight, it is definitely not a time for sex: get your problems straightened out first, emotionally, before you move on to anything physically.

The Secret of Sexual Communication

Sexual communication is a lot like regular communication: it uses the same ingredients as sharing emotional intimacy. Review Chapter Two: How to Treat A Girl Right, on the section about communication.

> Self Disclosure + Acceptance = Closeness

The same formula of talking, listening, and being accepting add up to closeness, except with sexual communication, you add in sexual thoughts and feelings to the conversation. In simple terms, when you talk openly about sex, and you both act accepting and supporting, then you will feel close and intimate with each other, sexually speaking.

One of the ways you might want to talk about sex as a couple, when you feel like you are comfortable and close enough, is take the Dr. Darcy's "Am I Ready for Sex?" Quiz in Chapter Four, together. Whether you are a virgin or you've already had sexual experiences, it's important that you are ready for sex with each new sexual partner, whether you are 14 years old or 74 years old! As a guy, you really do need to learn to talk to girls about sex, each and every time.

Last Minute Sex Test

Some guys fool themselves into believing that "sex is no big deal." Yet, when they look back, they realize it was, but they didn't expect to feel the way that the experience made them feel. Don't just let sex happen. Think about it first. If you are in the middle of a date, or in some other sudden sexual situation, try to answer these two last-minute questions when you are alone. If you are having doubts, make a quick escape to the bathroom, and give yourself a couple of minutes to think. Take a minute first, so you don't have second thoughts about the first time, or any time.

Quick Hit: Last Minute Sex Test

- How will I feel after sex with this person?
- How will I think about myself after sex?

What Teens Think About Before Sex

Emotionally, a lot of people feel very nervous before sex. Most teens have inadequate sexual communication, let alone every day communication skills. Even if you have a good relationship, it is hard to know what each other is thinking and feeling about before sex, especially on any given day. So, most teens have a lot of emotional insecurity about sex. Guys, even more than girls, do not usually express it because they are too embarrassed that they will look, feel or act inexperienced and stupid. If you have insecurities, you are not alone. Below are some of those fears and thoughts that many teens have, so you will know: What's on the mind, before sex?

Some Things Guys Think About Before Sex

- When guys have sex for the first time, they often think, "I feel a special connection and hope she feels a special connection, too!"

- "I'm afraid she might get pregnant!"

- "I just want to lose my virginity"—and nothing else matters but feeling the physical experience they have looked forward to for a long time.

- If you've have had sex before, with someone else, you may feel some of the same feelings as when you lost your virginity, but there can be less of the emotional connection with your girlfriend and more interest in the physical pleasures of sex.

- "Does she think I'm hot?"

- "What does she look like naked?"

- Some guys worry about their "performance," or if they will sexually please their girlfriend.

- Some guys are on the quest for making sure a girl has an orgasm.
- Some guys wonder if their penis is big enough (six inches is the average size, fully erect).
- Guys worry that they will ejaculate too soon. No one wants to be a "one-minute-man," or "premie," having premature ejaculation and come too quickly.
- Some guys want to make sex last too long, thinking it proves they're sexual stud-muffins, without realizing it might not be what a girl wants.
- Some guys may want to prove to themselves that they are not gay by having sex.
- Some guys just want to experience sexual control over another person.

Some Things Girls Think About Before Sex

- Girls worry that sex for the first time will be physically painful.
- Girls worry about pregnancy and STDs and they want protection. A lot of times, they are too afraid to talk about protection, and they want the guy to bring it up.
- Girls tend to need a lot of reassurance from a guy that they are loved and respected. It is important for a girl to feel like she did the right thing. She will know this by how a guy acts not only before sex but also after sex.
- Girls worry about their bodies and if they look good naked. They are worried about being too fat, if their breasts are attractive or too big or too small, if their stomach is flat, or if their butt is OK.

- Girls are afraid that they'll get pressured into sex and go farther than they want to go with sexual exploration.

- If sex "just happens" and they didn't talk to the guy about it ahead of time, they tend to have feelings of remorse, sadness, and guilt.

- It is always best for virgin sex to be planned. Girls need to talk about sex and be prepared, emotionally and physically, to share their virginity.

- Girls think about orgasms, although not so much the first time. They wonder if they will have one, how to have one, and what it is like.

- Girls think about the guy's orgasm. They wonder, when will he come and what will it be like? On giving oral sex, girls wonder what they're supposed to do when the guy comes: pull off, spit, or swallow? (Many girls expect a guy will not ejaculate in their mouth or he will pull out when he comes.)

- On getting oral sex, girls worry if they smell OK (because of all the tasteless jokes and advertisements for feminine hygiene products) and if their partner really wants to do it.

- Girls are not worried about the size of a man's penis, unless it really seems too big.

- Some girls get scared when they see an erect penis for the first time and wonder, "How is that big thing going to fit inside of me?"

- Girls want to make sure they are the "only one" and a guy is not just "playin' her" and using her for just sex.

- If a girl is having casual sex, she still wants to feel respected by the guy and know the guy will treat her like a friend afterwards.

PART II: THE PHYSICAL SIDE OF SEX

Secretly, the most important sexual question for guys is simply, "What do I do when I have sex?" One of the hidden truths of youth, is that young men want to learn to be good lovers, and they are afraid they will fail. All guys, especially being a virgin and inexperienced, wonder exactly what they are supposed to do, when it comes to the physical side of sex. Guys worry that it is very important for them to "perform," correctly or learn to be good at sex. This section of the book is going to give you guidance on how to have sex for the first time, and beyond, so you won't be embarrassed, feel insecure, feel stupid, and most importantly, learn how to share pleasurable, enjoyable sex.

In truth, the secret is: there is no big secret to great sex, except to experience pleasure together. There is no right move or perfect position or exact action for sex. If you are caring, passionate, have enthusiasm, and patience, you will always be a great lover. If all else fails: share a hug, laugh, and remember it is all about sharing love, nothing more, nothing less.

First, we'll review the three rules of sex from Chapter Two, then begin with the three steps of virgin sex.

Sex Rules: The Three Rules of Sex

- Rule #1 Get permission
- Rule #2 If a girl says "No": STOP
- Rule #3 No pain—EVER

Rule #1: Permission

Permission means that a girl needs says yes to sex, whether it is for kissing, hugging, making out, sexual touch or sexual intercourse. Permission means each partner has to say yes to sex every time.

Permission means permission to experiment with sexual experiences that may occur at different times on different occasions in different ways on different days.

================

> Permission means hearing "yes," from your sexual partner every step of the way.

================

Rule #2: If a girl says "No": STOP

Simply, no matter what, if a girl says no, stop. This rule is true whether you are a teenager, or whether you are a grown man. Sometimes a girl says "no," because she is in pain, and you need to talk and adjust and do something else, but no matter what, you need to stop. Sometimes a girl says no because she changes her mind, because she feels uncomfortable. Sometimes a girl says no and she doesn't know why, she just wants to stop or do something different. Work together, change, but no matter what, stop at that time.

233

Rule #3: No pain—EVER

Whether you are a teenager or a grown man, when you are with a sexual partner, one of the important sexual rules is to never have sexual pain. Sex is about sexual pleasure and sharing sexual joy and sharing love. Physically, sex can be very pleasurable, but at times, in certain circumstances, positions, places, or with actions, sex can cause physical discomfort. When there is sexual discomfort, you need to stop, no matter what. You can certainly continue later, when the pain subsides, after you find out what is wrong, but until then, you need to stop. In most situations, this will take a minor adjustment. At some times, it means that one sexual act will stop, but most of the time, loving and caring can continue with holding and touching.

THE THREE STEPS OF SEX

The urban sexual myth is that guys will know what to do, they're the "experienced" ones and that they'll have control over sex. Guys usually don't know what they are doing any more than girls! The myth needs to be replaced with some practical guidance, so this next section will teach you about the three steps of sex. If you have had previous sexual experiences, but you have not yet experienced sexual intercourse, then you will be familiar with some of the experiences in steps one and two, from talking to sexual touch. Even if you've had some previous sexual experience, you will probably learn new things about sex you may never have thought of before.

Most teens believe the myth that virgin sex will physically hurt the girl. Girls are often nervous and afraid of sex for the first time. The three steps of virgin sex will guide you, as a guy, step by step, on how to have sex with a girl. Also, it will guide you on having sex with a girl who is a virgin, without her having physical pain. Whether you are having sex for the first time or for the 1,000th time, taking things one step at a time, using the three steps of sex, will work every time.

The Three Steps of Virgin Sex

1. Talking and Listening
2. Touching and Feeling
3. Sexual Touch and Sexual Intercourse

Talking and Listening

Talking and listening is the first step of virgin sex. If you have read Chapter Two: Guys and Lies: How to Treat a Girl Right, you should have had a chance to learn about communication with girls.

Communication is the first step of sex, with general communication and then, sexual communication, before you choose to be sexually active, ideally. Sexual touch has to be negotiated, as you go along. This means you need to be talking about what you like and what you don't like with touch before you begin to touch each other, especially with sexual touch.

The truth is, most couples don't talk a lot about what they like with sexual touch before they simply start kissing and making out. They just start kissing and touching each other and if it feels right, they continue. Yet, sometimes, the kissing is too hard, or the touch is a little uncomfortable and even minor adjustments need to be made, even in the beginning. Let's say you want to kiss your girlfriend in your parked car. You lean way over to give her a big bear hug and kiss, you're enjoying a passionate long French kiss, steaming up with windows, and you think she is enjoying it too. Meanwhile, her back is shoved up against the door and it's killing her. Believe it or not, some girls are too afraid to tell you to stop and sit up a little bit, so her back won't have a dent it in the size of a door handle, so she can kiss you back comfortably! You have to be able to speak up with each other and not be too nervous to say something, fearing it might "ruin the moment" or you'll "say the wrong thing." Spend enough time with each other before you move on to sex, so that you know you can have a sexual voice and say what you're thinking or feeling. Learn to laugh about little things, like, "Hey, Casanova, your kiss is great, but my back is about to break in half!"

> If you're comfortable talking and listening to each other, so you aren't worried you'll hurt each other's feelings over small things, then you will be ready to move on to the next step of Virgin Sex.

Touching and Feeling

Touching and feeling is the second step of virgin sex. A physical relationship starts with touch. Some sex therapists consider the skin the largest sex organ, since it covers your whole body. Touch is very powerful physically and emotionally, but it is largely overlooked as it relates to sexual experience unless there is genital contact.

Touch can be very exciting and erotic, but if it does not include sexual contact, most guys don't think of it as sex. For example, kissing can be fun, hot, passionate, intimate, and sexy, but it's not considered sexual, since no sexual parts are touched. Yet, for a lot of girls and guys, lots of touching, like deep kissing, making out, or even back rubs, are big turn-ons, and essential parts of foreplay. Learn to be affectionate in an ongoing way, in little ways, like kissing her on the back of the neck when you're out for a walk. Touch her face, while you look at her straight in the eye when you're in public and tell her something you like about her. Touch her unexpectedly on the hand while she is talking to you. Do that thing they do in the movies when the man grabs the girl, backs her against the wall and kisses her, while moving his hand up her leg. Girls really do go for that stuff. Touch can be a lot of fun. Be playful. Be imaginative. Be yourself.

The most important part of this step of physical sharing is for you to experience and feel comfortable with physical touch. First, enjoy being physical with a girl in a safe, non-threatening way, which means she's not going to pressure you and you're not going to pressure her for sexual touch or sex. You need to become comfortable with touching before sexual touching. Allow yourself to simply experience the pleasure and joy of touch with your girlfriend.

Guys and Touch

The truth is that most teenage guys have very little touch in their lives! Girls often touch and hug each other. Mothers and daugh-

236

ters hug each other. Girls sleep over at each other's houses and lay around on each other's couches and share the same beds. Girls even all get out of the car and go to the bathroom together. Guys don't do this! Guys might get an occasional hug from their mom or dad, some don't. Guys might get a pat on the arm or butt in football practice, most don't. The reality is this: guys are often not very comfortable with the simple act of touching when they are teenagers! This is one of the reasons guys are so "awkward" when it comes to girls. It is not just that you guys don't know how to talk to girls, or that you are afraid to ask girls out, or that you don't know what to do when it comes to sex and you're supposed to be the expert. The truth is, after years of minimal touch, it is no wonder it is "awkward" for guys to be physically affectionate with girls. Learning to be comfortable with touch again is an important part of being a sexual person.

Being Uncomfortable with Touching

If you don't feel comfortable with your partner with non-sexual touch, don't go any farther, until you figure out what is wrong. When things don't feel right, it is very confusing. At this point, a lot of guys make an excuse and leave suddenly. One minute a couple is making out, the next minute, a guy bolts. This leaves everyone wondering what happened.

- It may be that you just need practice overcoming the newness of being with a girl.
- It might be that be that you just don't have that "feeling" with this particular girl.
- You might need to make minor changes and start communicating.
- A girl is too aggressive and goes faster than you want.

If this girl is someone that is important to you or with whom you hope to share a sexual relationship, practice sharing your thoughts and feelings, until it feels right. If it never feels right, then don't move on to sex. Touching and feeling is the stage at which you decide if you want to have a more serious physical relationship or if you're compatible. It is really important to learn how to handle these uncomfortable moments that happen with touching and feeling. You can run away from it or you can face it. It seems to be the male coyote instinct to run. However, when you have the human maturity to face it, then you will know you are more "emotionally ready" for sex. While you can have sex without having sexual communication, you are setting yourself up for problems, sooner or later. Or you have to learn to trust each other as a couple to be prepared to talk about your feelings about touch and later, sex.

Sometimes, some girls can get aggressive, especially girls who are more experienced, or girls who want to prove something to you, like they want you to be their boyfriend or have future expectations or play games. All sexual touch between people needs to be negotiated and agreed upon. If you don't feel comfortable or you don't want to do anything: DON'T. Please know that when you go farther with a girl to sexual touch, remember, there might be Sex-pectations (see Chapter Four), even if you have sex just to have sex *for her*.

Foreplay

One of the most frequently asked sexual questions by teen guys is, "What *exactly* is foreplay?" Most guys have heard, "A girl likes to have a lot of foreplay before sex." Physically, foreplay involves non-sexual touch, including kissing, hugging, caressing, and making out BEFORE sexual touch or sexual intercourse. The second stage of virgin sex, touching and feeling, is included in a lot of definitions of foreplay. Some girls also consider some sexual touch foreplay, including breast fondling and oral sex, but generally foreplay is considered touching prior to sex that leads to sex.

Guys often want to go straight to "The Main Event": SEX. Girls want to take time to build up to sex, with touching and feeling, to build up sexual desire and sexual feelings, before they feel like having sexual touch and sex. This is true of younger and older women. Young women often say, they like to feel like they "make love all day long, then make love." As men get older, much older, they also desire more touch and foreplay, but most teenage boys do not require or desire much foreplay to want sex. It takes patience and maturity for guys to wait, and focus on pleasing, pleasure, and foreplay, many times for the sake of girls, before sexual touch and sexual play. Since you are making love with girls, and young women, listen to what they say. If they are happy and if they desire sex, it is more likely that they will want you, and want to make love with you. When you are wanted, when you feel comfortable with touch, when you feel sexual desire between you, you may choose to move to the next stage of sex: sexual touch and sexual intercourse.

239

Sexual Touch and Sexual Intercourse

Sexual touch and sexual intercourse is the third step of virgin sex. Finally, we're at the step most of you have been waiting for: sex. Remember: Losing your virginity is not a race. Unlike a sporting event, virgin sex is not an event, it is process, a process of sharing sexual pleasure with another person. Most guys are so curious about sex and biologically driven to desire sex and culturally driven to want to discover what sex is about, that they feel like they are in a race against time to lose their virginity and have sex the first chance they get. On that first run, there's the race to the finish line.

Let me remind you that sex is not an individual sport. You are with another person: A girl, a woman, a person you care about, your girlfriend, the person you love, maybe your wife. If you would like a repeat performance, you might like to know a few things about making love with a person. While most guys fantasize about what the physical sensations will be like, they also do, indeed worry about what moves they will make, how to please their partners, or to really be a good lover. This section of the book will give you detailed information about sexual touching, oral sex, anal sex, and sexual intercourse.

Sexual Touch

Sexual touch is the fun part, where you get to turn on the sexual wiring switch. The most important part of this step is to first have physical touch and exploration of each other's genitals, breasts, and buttocks, without sexual intercourse. You will want to explore what feels good to you and your partner with sexual touching, and also practice sexual communication before you move on to sexual intercourse. Remember, the three rules of sex all apply here, including asking for permission to touch a girl in a sexual area, be it her breasts, buttocks, or genitals, and she needs to ask you what is OK, too. At any point, you are responsible for asking for sexual touch and how much. Many guys, when they are making the moves, don't ask. If she doesn't say no, they take this as a "yes," and keep going. If she moves his hand away, he tries again, hoping she won't move it away again, then tries again, hoping she won't move it again, until he finally gives up or she gets up and or says "stop."

Sexual touch is tricky. How are you supposed to stop and ask for permission to sexually touch someone? C'mon, in the movies, they are just making out, fall on the bed, start ripping off each other's clothes, and the scene ends. The next thing you know, everyone knows they had sex, right? The tricky part is that no one really tells you how it happens in real life: negotiating about sexual touch never seems to happen, does it? This is the part about being a guy that can be tough. Yet, it's easy to learn to how to be very successful with sexual touch with girls, how to talk to them, and how to learn to touch, if you know the secret.

The Secret of Successful Sexual Touch

The secret of sexual touch for guys is to take touch one step at a time, to build sexual trust one step at a time, as you explore each other's bodies, as a process, not an event. The most important part of this secret is to build trust so that a girl can feel comfortable enough to get excited and sexually aroused, which will lead, in many cases, to her wanting to have sexual touch.

Successful sexual touch does not happen in one moment or on one day, it happens over time. Sometimes that time is several days or several weeks or several months or perhaps never. It is very, very important that when sexual touch occurs and it is right, and then one of you wants to slow down and stop, then you stop. It may be that you climb to the peak of excitement together, and you move down, then you climb back up, and then down, and maybe you are never quite reaching that goal of sex that you, as a guy have in mind, or that certain sexual touch, that you want at that moment, but you are building a foundation of trust, so that she knows she can enjoy sexual touch with you, and you can go together, safely.

Starting Talk About Sexual Touch

- Is this OK?
- Is it alright if I take off your top?
- Can I take off your bra?
- Can I touch your (breasts, butt, thighs, back)?
- Does that feel good?
- Is that alright?

The beginning of sexual touch is to start with touching non-genitally, with her breasts, buttocks, and body. Don't overlook the overall sexual touch of the body that doesn't include genital touching. Lightly touching the skin under the bra can be very sexy. Running your fingers down the spine can send chills all over the body. Think of touching her in a way with your imagination that she has not been touched and you would like to touch her. In turn, she can start by her touching your body, too. You might want to start with being dressed first, and then eventually discuss becoming undressed with each other, if and when you feel more comfortable with each other. Check in with each other about how you both feel, along the way, and on different days, over time. Are you both enjoying each other? Do you feel excited? Do you feel passion and sexual excitement? Remember to be caring and considerate of her feelings.

A Note on Breast Touching

- First, you might want learn how to take off a bra, smoothly. Most bras have back hooks, but some are hooked in the front. A very smooth move is when a guy knows how to un-hook a bra, without fumbling with a hook for an extended period of time. If it's a sports bra, forget it: they come off over the head.

- Second, pause and look. Make a compliment before you touch, not grab.

- Third, start by touching the outside of the breast, not the nip-ple. Generally, the outside of the breast is not tender, even if the girl is on her period or even if she has tender or sensitive nipples, so you'll be "safe."

- Fourth, gently touch the nipples. Most girls do not like to have their nipples pinched, at least at this level of sexual touch.

Most guys gets excited, included getting sexually aroused, from just a little sexual touch. Don't worry about having a erection, but try not to physically press it into her; girls can get turned off by feeling your erection, at least initially. Don't worry about getting excited or getting "blue balls." If you get aroused, you can always go home and masturbate, without putting any expectations and pressure on her. Remember, when you masturbate later, the excitement that you share together will follow you later, while the "pressure," that you feel will be released, without putting it on your relationship.

Once you feel comfortable with the beginning of sexual touch, which, again, can take time, often weeks or months in a relationship, then talk about moving on to sexual touch, including genital touch. If you want to have sexual touch with a girl, whether she wants to keep her virginity or not, she must simply like you and trust you.

> Some guys think that they have to convince a girl to have sex or pressure her for sex or threaten to break up with her to have sex. These are the moves of immature, amateurish, selfish boys!

When a girl likes you and trusts you and enjoys your touch, you will not have to convince a girl to want you. When you kiss and touch and love and care for a girl and treat her right, while keeping your relationship discrete (read: keep quiet about your physical relationship), *she will be asking you to touch her.*

Girls and Virginity

Many girls are afraid to have sexual touch, because they are afraid it will lead to losing their virginity. Many girls want to keep their virginity and they are afraid any sexual touch will lead to sex. Girls have some very good reasons for not wanting to have sex. One very big reason is that a lot of girls want to wait until they are married to have sex. About one in five girls, even in the 21st century, is still a virgin when she marries. Another reason is a fear of pregnancy.

Another might be that she is waiting until she is older, or for any other reasons that are her "conditions" for sex.

Many girls are still interested in sharing sexual touch, even though they are often very concerned about not being ready for sexual intercourse. In order to agree to having sexual touch, she would have to trust the guy a lot, and know that he wouldn't pressure her to have sexual intercourse, nor force her to have sex. Fear of being forced or coerced into sex is a very real concern for girls. About one in 10 girls is date raped, meaning she is in a "date situation" with a guy who forces her to have sex with him, even though she said no. Also, some girls are afraid that if they lead a guy on, and he gets really excited, he won't control himself, and it will be her fault. So some girls avoid situations with a guy where he could take advantage of her. Again, overcoming this fear is easy when you take things slow and show her that she can trust you completely.

Genital touching of girls

Before a girl is ready for intercourse sex, an exploration of her sexual parts, and discovering her sexual response, is essential. Ideally, as stated earlier, a girl should have some personal sexual skills before trying to have sexual intercourse, including finding out what she likes sexually and how she responds to sexual touch and even how to bring herself to orgasm. If a girl knows nothing about herself and sexual touch, it is going to be up to you, as a couple to explore genital touching, together. As a guy, you can help her by being encouraging, patient, and helping her discover how she responds to sexual touch.

For girls, usually the most sexually exciting part of her body is her clitoris. The sensitivity of the clitoris is similar to sensitivity of the tip of a man's penis, but even more so, in a concentrated area. Most inexperienced guys don't know where a clitoris is or how to touch it. The clitoris is located just below the pubic bone and above the urethra opening, under a layer of skin, called the "clitoral hood." The clitoral hood varies in size among women, but women almost always have sensitivity of feeling through touching of the clitoris. Typically, most girls, dressed or naked, will experience sexual pleasure with touch to the clitoris. Clitoral touch can be with a leg, pelvis, hand, vibrator, mouth, or tongue. Generally, clitoral stimulation involves rubbing a clitoris with a finger or two in an up and down, back and forth, or with a pressing motion, depending on what she likes. You can encourage your partner to use her sexual voice and give you directions. She can start by telling you: higher, lower, faster, slower, softer, or harder. In some cases, you might put your hand on hers and let her guide you with the motions that are pleasurable and exciting to her. Most girls will feel sexually aroused from clitoral stimulation.

Sexual arousal is different for girls and guys. Guys know when they are sexual excited and aroused: their erection is standing hard in front of them. Girls, believe it or not, don't always know if they are excited or turned on. A lot of girls don't know how to get aroused. Some girls get turned on from simply kissing, hugging, or touching. Most girls may need more direct clitoral stimulation with the touch of a hand or mouth. Some girls also have sexual arousal from sexual intercourse, which will be discussed later. Physically, there are some signs of arousal for girls: her vagina gets lubricated or "wet," sometimes her heart beats faster, sometimes there is a red flush on her chest, sometimes it is just a feeling of being "horny" or sexually excited. Most girls can have an orgasm from clitoral stimulation. See Chapter Six on sexual response and orgasms for a review. Remember: before a girl will be ready for sexual intercourse, she needs to know how to get excited and to be physically aroused to be ready for sex. Sometimes it takes a long time for girls to learn to feel comfortable with and respond to sexual touch. Often, girls may take weeks or months to learn how to become aroused enough to have an orgasm.

Genital touching of guys

Most of the time, guys need to be patient when it comes to girls touching them genitally. Most guys welcome and enjoy genital touch. Most guys have a lot of experience with self-touch, masturbation, sexual arousal and orgasms, through sometimes years of sexual solo practice. In this way, more guys are often sexually more experienced than girls by the time they are having teenage relationships. Guys are a lot more confident about how their body works and with having orgasms, from masturbation. Can you imagine never having sexually touched yourself and having someone else touch you and experience your first orgasm in front of someone? Often, this is the case with girls! So, a guy needs to be patient with a girl, when it comes to sex. First, some girls have never even seen a penis before, if they are a virgin, or sexually inexperienced. Some girls are nervous about seeing a guy naked. Don't push yourself on a girl. If she is hesitant about touching you, genitally, at first, don't start by getting undressed in front of her. Keep your boxers on. Start with the basics: touching and feeling, lying down together with clothes on, and hugging. Let her feel you against her in an indirect way, in a casual way, when you are hugging or naturally pressed against each other. Don't press your penis in to her intentionally, wait until she is far more comfortable with you before you introduce your sexual self to your relationship. When you get more comfortable with touching and feeling, eventually, you will be hugging each other, at first fully clothed, and when you're making out, it gradually happens that your hugging becomes closer and tighter, and sooner rather than later, you will experience an erection when your are very close together. Sometimes, this kind of genital touching through clothing leads to erotic feelings and arousal and even dry humping (see below).

Eventually, if and when you get to the point that you are undressing and naked with each other, you can begin to share sexual touching. As with girls, sexual touch with a guy may start with a hand. First, you

246

can ask your partner to touch your penis. You may guide a girl to show her how you like to be touched or stroked. Start slow at first. You aren't starting by showing her how to give you a hand job to orgasm. Sexual touching at first is just for exploring and sharing feelings together. Let her explore your testicles and penis with her hand, and then later, with her mouth, and her tongue. Let her touch you in the way she would like to touch you at first, just for her pleasure and experience of discovery. Later, you may show her how to more vigorously stroke your penis using the type of motions that are pleasurable to you.

Oral Sex

Currently, oral sex is a very popular type of non-intercourse sex between teenagers. Oral sex is touching someone's genitals with your mouth, and it is also called "a blow job," or "getting head" (See Chapter Six for other slang). A recent national study on sex showed that 50% of 15 to 19 year olds engaged in oral sex, with both girls and boys equally giving and receiving oral sex (Mosher, Chandra, Jones, 2002). A lot of girls and guys don't seem to think that oral sex "counts" as sex, but if you are having sexual touch of any kind, it's sex. For guys and girls, please remember that oral sex is a risky sexual behavior, since it involves the transmission of sexual fluids from the genitals to the mouth (see Chapter Eight on STDs). One of the benefits of oral sex is that you can share love and intimacy and you will not get pregnant, and you can keep your virginity intact. Also, you can share a very intimate, exciting, and sexually fulfilling connection, that includes sexual orgasm.

Some guys put pressure on girls to give them oral sex if the girl doesn't want to have sexual intercourse. Putting pressure on girls because you are making someone responsible for your own sexual pressure is wrong. You are responsible for your own sexual needs, not a girl. Generally speaking, girls don't put pressure on guys to give them oral sex, but it can happen. Often, if guys are pressured, it is because they fear being ridiculed. Pressure for any kind of sex should be walked away from.

Anal Sex

Anal sex refers to sexual contact with the anus, which is commonly referred to as your "butthole." Anal sex can involve any stimulation of the anus, including touching, licking, or anal penetration. For some people, the anus is a highly sensitive area, bringing intense sexual pleasure, although many people feel "grossed out" by any anal contact. Touching may include touching with a hand or an object, such as tickling with a feather. Anal touching with a mouth may be as simple as kissing and touching the area around the anus. Actually licking the anus for sexual play is called "rimming." Rimming is unsafe sex, and a latex barrier or part of a condom needs to be used to have safer sex.

A lot of guys have sexual fantasies about anal sex. Many guys want to try to have anal sex with their girlfriends or wives, at one time or the other. Most girls do not want to try anal sex. Some girls have already tried anal sex and many found it hurt and have no interest in trying it again. For some girls, few, but some, anal sex is *the* type of sex that they enjoy.

Anal penetration needs to begin very slowly, or it will probably be the first and last experience with anal sex you will ever have with that particular partner. The opening of the anus has a sphincter, which is less elastic than a vagina, which means it is very tight. Anal penetration can be very painful, unless one is physically ready for it, and many people never get used to it, nor want to. You need to learn relaxation, and you need a lot of lubrication. For most people, it takes days, weeks, or months for the anal sphincter to stretch out and be prepared for anal penetration. Anal penetration can begin with a tongue or finger, and may progress to using a small, slender object or anal dildo, or a penis.

Some teenagers choose to engage in anal sex for experimentation, to enjoy sexual variation and pleasure, or to have sexual intercourse during a woman's period; but one of the biggest reasons for teenagers to have anal sex is to avoid the risk of pregnancy that accompanies vaginal intercourse. It is important to know that anal sex still carries the risk of STDs, especially Hepatitis B, and all sexual precautions need to be taken. Some people never learn to enjoy anal sex and/or have no interest in this type of sexual experimentation, however. Anal sex, or "buggery" as it used to be called, is illegal in several states.

Dry Humping (Dry Sex or Frottage)

Dry humping is a form of "outercourse," or sex without having sexual penetration. Dry humping is like simulated intercourse, with your clothes on, which interestingly, is often repeated even in adult life from time to time. This includes rubbing against each others' genitals in sexual motions, pressing hard against each other, that is sexually arousing. The sexual positions used can be simply one on top of the other, or it may be in a sexual "scissors" position, where both partner's legs are straddled with each other. In the dry humping movements, each partner can rub and grind erotically with each other, providing sexual arousal and often experiencing orgasm, without the risk of pregnancy, and keeping virginity intact. Often, dry humping involves clitoral orgasms for girls and blue balls for guys.

SEXUAL INTERCOURSE

Sexual intercourse is the last step of virgin sex. After almost 9 chapters, 3 rules of sex, the emotional parts of sex, and the first two steps of virgin sex, you finally have arrived at sexual intercourse. Funny, but when most guys think of sex, they think of sexual intercourse

FIRST. Sad, but true, that to have great sex, you've got to think of all of the other things first, if you're going to get to sex, now and for the rest of your life. This may not sound fair, but it is the way that it is. The good news is that if you are willing to take the time to do things right from the beginning, it is more likely that the girl you are with will learn to enjoy and love to share sex with you. After you begin slowly, things tend to heat up quickly over time. When you have the right start, the right foundation, you can have a great time together as lovers, sometimes for many years.

The truth is, a woman needs to have emotional sexual desire first, then physical arousal, then sexual play before sexual intercourse. Intercourse is reserved only for a moment in time when both partners first and foremost feel completely comfortable with the sexual pleasuring. Sexual intercourse, like sexual touch, is a process, not an event, that often requires several days of preparation in order to avoid physical pain the first time, when you have sex with a virgin. Even if you are having sex with someone who is sexually experienced, girls still need to have foreplay and be physically aroused to enjoy sexual intercourse every time.

Why Is It So Important for a Girl to be "Wet"?

When a girl is sexually excited, her vagina gets lubricated or "wet." When girls get aroused, their vaginas get moist and their vaginas expand: the vaginal walls get thicker and expand in length, making the penetration of a finger or penis possible. A girl's vagina often expands about 2 inches in length during arousal. The average girl's vagina is 4 inches in length, which means when she is aroused, it expands to 6 inches. The average length of a man's erect penis is also 6 inches in length. So, when a girl is sexually aroused, it allows her to accommodate the average size of a man's penis. If a girl has sex with a guy when she is not physically aroused, when her vaginal length is only 4 inches and his penis length is 6 inches, sexual intercourse will cause sexual pain. With a lack of sexual arousal, a man's penis during sexual thrusting will hit against the woman's cervix (at the end of her vagina), which a man will feel, and it will hurt the woman. Hence, it is very, very important that a woman be sexual aroused to be able to have enjoyable sex.

Sexual intercourse with virgins: opening the hymen

Prior to sexual intercourse, after "foreplay" or sexual touch, using a gentle finger to first experience vaginal penetration is the best way to prepare for pain-free, comfortable, and pleasurable sexual intercourse. A virgin girl's vagina has a thin layer of skin, called the hymen, which is at the entrance of her vagina. If you are having sex with a girl who is a virgin, her hymen needs to be gently opened. Sometimes, by the time a young woman has intercourse, her hymen is already opened, from exercise or accidents, but girls also have an "emotional hymen" or their emotion opening to sex, as well as a real physical need to have her vagina slowly introduced to sex. Even when a young woman has not had intercourse for a long time, her vagina can be too tight for penetration, and she will need to very slowly experience vaginal penetration.

Think of the process of opening the vagina as almost motionless.

A finger is much smaller, and less scary and intimidating, than a penis for most girls, for initial vaginal penetration. Using your finger as a guide, gently insert your fingers inside the vagina, at first with very little movement at all. Ever so slowly, the vaginal opening can be stretched, until your finger can comfortable be placed into the vagina. Slowly progress to moving your finger side to side, up to an inch in width, and in and out, until you reach the end of her vagina. During this sexual play, if any discomfort is experienced at all, stop immediately. Return to pleasurable touching, including kissing, fondling, sexual touch, and clitoral stimulation to increase sexual arousal.

Sexual arousal decreases sexual pain. When a woman is experiencing sexual arousal and excitement and pleasure, she does not feel the sensations of discomfort or sexual pain, in the same way as in a relaxed state. So, when you are in the process of opening a virgin girl's hymen, it is very important that this occurs only when she is very sexually excited, so she will not experience any or at least, only a minimal of physical discomfort. Often, this process of getting excited, sharing sexual play, trying a little bit of inserting your finger into her vagina, then stopping, then starting again, then getting aroused again, then stopping, can take place over a period of hours, or days or even weeks. Remember, this is not a race. Opening the hymen can take some time, it might be unusually thick, and there might be some bleeding and slight discomfort. However, if you follow this process slowly, often women experience little or no pain, they might feel excitement and pleasure, and they will soon be ready to experience sexual intercourse with a penis. Prior to beginning intercourse, a girl should be very sexually aroused, so be sure to share sexual touching, including kissing, clitoral play, caressing, and oral sex, or whatever you have found to be sexually arousing for foreplay prior to penetration with the penis.

Prior to entering her vagina for sexual intercourse, your penis needs to be erect and lubricated. (If you are also a virgin, see below, first.) You should be wearing a condom, and you can use the lubricant on a condom, or use saliva, so that you can slide easily into her vagina. It is often helpful if she can hold your penis with her hand and guide it in slowly to the opening of her vagina, although you should also be able to find the opening, by this time. At first, put just the head of your penis inside her: that is all. You are not looking to have sexual intercourse with thrusting at this point: only to have your penis inside her vagina and to not move. Don't worry right away about moving or performing, just focus on how it feels to be inside her vagina. Make sure that her vagina is always lubricated and moist for comfortable penetration. If necessary, for the first few days, alternate between penetration on one day with your penis and the next with your finger to stretch out her vagina and prepare for full sexual intercourse. Also, don't limit your lovemaking to intercourse: continue kissing, touching, looking into each other's eyes, and feeling other parts of each other's bodies. For one thing, you want to stay excited, aroused and hard, but you also want to share affection and love.

Sexual intercourse for the first time, with a virgin, often needs to take place very slowly over a few days or weeks, just in case the hymen is not fully opened, which may require a gentle push, eventually. If she is able to have orgasms, have sexual play first, having an orgasm first, then becoming aroused again, followed by sexual intercourse, as it is more likely that she will be able to have greater penetration with a penis after full sexual arousal. Once full penetration is possible, you can begin to slowly move your penis in and out of her vagina without your penis completely leaving her vagina. Take your time with increasing the speed and depth of thrusting. For the first several times that you have sexual intercourse, up to the first ten or twelve times, you need to take it slowly, as the vagina may be sore from the hymen tearing and repairing itself, or stretching out for the first time.

Virgin Sex for Guys

Whether you are with a girl who is a virgin or a girl who is sexually experienced, most of the rules and steps above apply, except the last few paragraphs. If you are not with a virgin, you will not have to be as careful about vaginal penetration. In every case, with every girl, on every occasion, every woman needs to be physically aroused to be ready for sex. However, with sexually experienced women, the average woman takes 8 minutes to get aroused and ready for sex vs. days, weeks, or months for the average virgin. Why guys fantasize about virgins is a mystery to me!

Most guys have very different feelings, thoughts, and desires about sex than girls, especially when it comes to sex for the first few times. While girls are worried about the emotional parts of sex, guys tend to be much more concerned with the physical parts of sex. Most guys want to know what the physical experience will be like: what she will feel like, what it will feel like to be inside of her, what it will feel like to come.

The One-Second Wonder—Jarod's Story

The first time, Jarod waited for 6 months for his girlfriend to be ready for sex. They were waiting until after her junior prom. It was his senior prom. They rented a hotel room. It was supposed to be the most romantic night of their life. She wanted her first time to be really special for her. He really wanted it to be special for her. So, he waited 3 months after he first asked her to have sex, until the prom, to make her first time right for her.

They had done "everything together sexually" but have sexual intercourse, so they both knew each other really well. They both really loved each other, too.

Prom night came. Neither of them had anything to drink before prom, and they waited until after the prom, until they got to their room, away from all of their friends, for their long, hot night of prom sex (Jarod laughs at this part of the story.)

They got undressed.

Wow! Jarod said Bianca just looked so beautiful! She had on this hot, sexy, new thong and bra, and she just looked so gorgeous!

They got in bed. They kissed. They were making out. Bianca was ready for sex. Jarod made sure she was wet and ready to go! He slowly started to put his penis inside her, not wanting to hurt her and making sure she was fine, and, it just felt so good, that he lost his breath. All the breath in his lungs disappeared. All the air in the room was gone. He tried to find it, because he knew if he couldn't, he was going to come right then and it would be over, their long awaited moment, in one second.

Boom.

It was over.

Yep, after all that waiting, it was over in one second.

There was a very awkward silence.

Jarod was very embarrassed.

Bianca laughed and said, "Soooo, am I still a virgin?

Then, Jarod laughed, too. "Hopefully, not for long."

Jarod said, "Here, we had this room, for the whole night, that I paid $100 for and we sat in bed and watched movies all night long. It was still one of the funnest nights of my life, but she wasn't a virgin when she woke up."

The truth is, most guys get so excited the first time, that they will want to "go for it" and . . . it's over. It might be best to simply think of your first time as "my first moment." The first time is not about performing, it is about the experience. For Jarod, his first time was, "the funnest night of his life!"

Think about your first sexual experiences as your simply first experiencing being with someone, seeing how it feels physically to feel new physical sensations, and to let go of expectations of how long you last or how you might perform as a lover. For most guys, it is very difficult to control your ejaculation the first few times you have sex. It is very easy to get excited and come very quickly, sometimes even before sexual penetration happens. If you come very quickly and have premature ejaculation, it is a very normal part of first sexual experiences. The first time, you might want to consider just trying to experience vaginal penetration, without moving, at first. First, simply experience sexual penetration. If you don't come immediately, move slowly. The second time, again, think about just having vaginal penetration, don't focus on moving, and enjoy the sensation with just staying still. As a young man, if you initially have a rapid ejaculation, your partner may be willing to try again, just wait a few minutes, try again and usually on the second time, you will last a little longer, but you should still focus on moving slowly at first, rather than fast and hard. Most important, if you come more quickly than you would like, which is more than likely to happen, don't worry about it, it is perfectly normal part of the experience of really enjoying sex.

If things go "wrong" and nothing seems to be clicking together once in a while, don't worry about it and don't blame each other. Just as with anything in life, timing can be off, unpredictable events interrupt you, and you can change your mood. The important thing to remember is that sex is about sharing love, and if you start and continue with talking and listening, you can work this situation out. If you and your partner work together to make virgin sex right, sex can be a lifelong pleasure, filled with intimacy and love, and more sex.

P.S. How do you know if a girl is really enjoying sex?

You can guess or you can ask. Of course, you can make an educated guess. Most guys think they know when a girl has had an orgasm, and that, of course, is the sign that a girl had a good time, right? First of all, a girl doesn't have to have an orgasm to really enjoy sex. She might be having a really great time, the best time of her life, but she just didn't have an orgasm. Or maybe she had five orgasms, but she didn't like you. Remember, not all girls have orgasms: most girls have orgasms from clitoral stimulation, some from rubbing, during intercourse, and only 50% of girls have orgasms from intercourse alone. So, how do you know?

In the movie, *When Harry Met Sally*, Billy Crystal tells Meg Ryan that he knows for sure when a girl has an orgasm. Meg Ryan proves to him that a girl can fake an orgasm, by faking one, right in the middle of a restaurant, on the big movie screen. It was convincing: Women can and do fake orgasms. Why? Women fake it because sometimes they can't have an orgasm or they don't feel like having one and when they don't want their partners to continue having sex, they fake it, so a guy will finish. That is sad. A girl shouldn't have to fake an orgasm to end sex or to prove to you that you're a good lover. She should have an orgasm because she feels like it. Period.

Of course, you'd like her to get pleasure from sex. Most guys want to make sure their partner is getting pleasure. If you care, if you aren't sure, ask. Better than asking if she's had an orgasm, ask her if there is anything else she would like you to do for her. Even if she's had three orgasms, she might want one more, and she'll think you're a great lover, if you ask. Even if she's had a wonderful time with you and she's had no orgasms, she'll think you care. Either way, you win and so does she. That way, you will know if she is really enjoying sex.

AFTER SEX

OK, now you have thought about everything you think you need to consider before making a decision about having sex. Now what do you do after sex, to make sure everything is right for you and your partner? After making love for the first time, most girls and guys don't know the right things to say or do. They are not sure what to say when it comes to sharing emotional or physical feelings. Virgin sex is a sharing of a very special part of your being for the first time in your life. Many people experience a very deep emotional and physical closeness for the very first time in their lives. Yet, some people, especially those who don't have an emotional connection with their partner, don't feel much different and they wonder, "What's the big deal?" For almost all young men and women, this is a new kind of closeness that they have never experienced before, and they simply don't know what to do or say because they have never been in this situation. Here are guidelines to starting things off right.

The truth is, sexual closeness is different than almost anything you will experience in your life. It will change your relationship with your partner and your relationship with yourself forever. Good luck!

A Guy's After Sex Guide

- Right after you make love, stay together and cuddle.
- Don't just get up and leave.
- While you're still together, ask her if everything was OK for her. Tell her how it felt for you. Really listen to what she tells you about this experience and her feelings.
- Afterwards, always be in contact at least by the next day.
- Call her, talk to her, be nice. Tell her how much you appreciated making love.
- If you're in school or work together, seek her out first thing in the day and kiss and hug her, or just tell her how you feel, like you're glad to see her.
- Ask if she's OK.
- Send an e-mail, but don't only send an e-mail, and remember not all e-mail is private.
- Do not break up right afterward. Tell her you still love/like her and want to see her again, or explain why you can't see

her right away if this is the case. If the relationship proves not to be what you wanted, then explain this to her as well, letting her know that the sex was not the only reason you were with her in the first place.

- Tell her how you feel. This is not about how things were sexually, but about how things were emotionally, how you felt about her. Anyone can share what they felt in a particular moment, describing sexual sensations, but if you want to treat a girl right, tell her how you feel about her emotionally.

- Tell her what you liked about her physically. Be specific.

- Tell her what you think is beautiful about her: her eyes, her lips, her mouth, her kisses, her breasts, her hips, her smell, her taste.

- Tell her what you think about her laugh, the way she moved, or how beautiful her facial and body expressions were.

- Most importantly, contact her. Even if you are shy and don't know what to say, call her and tell her you enjoyed being with her. The simplest expression of caring will prevent a lot of emotional insecurity, questions, and pain.

- Reassure each other that this is a private thing, something you will keep between the two of you.

- Don't be a big mouth . . . and a big jerk. Don't go bragging to everyone and spreading rumors.

- Talk to your best friend, if you have one, *and* if you trust him or her to be private and keep their mouth shut!

- Don't expect sex again just because you did it once. Don't put the pressure on for more sex.

NINE

WHAT EVERY GUY NEEDS TO KNOW ABOUT PHYSICAL AND SEXUAL ABUSE

260

Tragically, abuse is a common experience for teens today. At least half of teens will experience or witness some type of abuse, from neglect to physical abuse, from sexual molestation to sexual abuse, from dating violence to date rape. Many boys experience childhood physical abuse and sexual abuse. In turn, many boys grow up to become violent men who abuse girls and women physically and sexually. By the time boys are teenagers, one out of three teen dating relationships experience violence.

Silence about violence is an emotional killer.

Abuse is a taboo subject, especially for boys, because they feel embarrassed or guilty about the abuse, especially when they are the victims of sexual abuse. Breaking the silence, especially the sexual silence on abuse, and giving guys guidance and resources for recovery is very important for themselves and in having healthy relationships with girls. Abuse can have devastating effects on a person's ability to have relationships, to trust people, and to see the world as a safe place in general. Physical, emotional, and sexual trauma can affect self esteem, mental health, sexuality, and how young men experience relationships and treat girls. Guys need to know how sex can be abusive, how to avoid such abuse, and what to do if it happens to them or a friend.

A few young men who have experienced different types of abuse courageously share their stories in this chapter. They tell how physical and sexual abuse happened to them and how it affected them, emotionally and sexually. Sexual abuse has many definitions, so these are summarized here for you. This chapter also talks about dating violence and date rape. Physical violence and date rape are serious problems in teen relationships. One in four girls is date raped in college, which is rape committed by an acquaintance or boyfriend, and 30% of teen relationships experience some type of violence. Rape and assault are illegal and wrong. Common myths and misconceptions about date rape, as well as understanding and avoiding the roots of violence in relationships are discussed.

Warning to teens and their parents: This chapter contains detailed information about physical and sexual abuse, rape, and young men's real stories of their experiences with trauma. While efforts have been made to prevent presenting this information in a sexually explicit manner, some of the content may be shocking and intense to young teenagers. While many teenagers may benefit from understanding physical and sexual abuse, younger teens may choose not to read the stories in this chapter.

PHYSICAL ABUSE

Broken Boys—Cap's Story

Cap remembers everything, including hiding under the bed, and having nightmares with flashes of violent pictures that still haunt his

sleep today. His parents split when he was 4, but he remembers what it was like before they separated. His father was very abusive to his mom—physically, mentally and emotional. Cap witnessed their fights many, many times.

Mom had affairs while she was married to his dad. His dad had affairs, too. His mom would take the kids with her to go and stay with other men, using the kids as a cover. Cap remembers sleeping over in strange men's houses, with his older sister and brother and his younger brother, sleeping on sleeping bags and waking up on strange couches. He would hear her with her boyfriends and walk in on them sometimes, naked and in intimate positions. He was confused. His older sister taught him to keep his mouth shut, or he'd see more beatings. When they got home, the fights and beatings would begin anyway.

His mom was always nurturing and protective to Cap, and he knew she loved him. She would hold him and draw him close to her chest, where he felt safe and secure. Yet, at times, she would run-away to her mother's house, across the street, but leaving Cap with his daddy. He was scared of his Daddy. When Cap was 5, his father took him and his little brother and ran away from his mom. Cap's daddy was the same daddy as his younger brother, but his older brother and sister had different dads. Cap's dad moved them about an hour away. His parents divorced and they had joint custody, but his dad got physical custody: probably because of lies he told about his mom. Lies he heard for the next 10 years of his life.

Cap's father was a womanizer, which meant he was always chasing women, wooing them with flowers and a fake charm that attracted a string of women, but sickened Cap. Cap's mom was his dad's second wife, of five altogether. Daddy was always gone working, drinking, and spending time and money on women. Cap and his brother sometimes had babysitter, sometimes they were left alone to fend for themselves, eating a lot of cereal and beans and rice.

Daddy started abusing Cap like he abused his mother. He started right off where he left off with his mom. At first, it was mental abuse. When Cap acted up, doing normal things that kids do, like jumping on a couch or fighting with his brother, his father would tell him he "was just like his mother!" His dad would degrade his mother, trying to alienate him from his mom, saying "she's horrible, she's a whore, she abandoned you, she never loved you, and she doesn't want you." Then his dad would try to keep him in line by threatening to send him back to his mother, threatening him by saying "she will throw you out on the streets and let you starve and abandon you. Keep being bad and I'll throw you off to her." Strangely, Cap never bought it. He was definitely afraid of his dad, but he never bought the lies about his mom.

Then, the beatings began. Big Texan Daddy had a big "Country Belt," that was heavy leather with a row of metal wire that was weaved onto the top and a row of wire weaved into the bottom of the belt. When he was 7, 8, 9, and 10, he was told, "I'm going to beat the Devil out of you," and Cap would get hit repeatedly with the belt. The metal hit his buttocks, back and legs, leaving blisters, sores, and welts all over his backside, to the point of really not being able to sit down. Once, Cap even got hit with a bullwhip across his legs. Daddy also liked throwing things. Once, he threw a broom right through the wall, leaving a huge hole, then turned around saying, "look what you made me do—hurry up and fix it!" Daddy was a violent man. He burned down two houses and burned up a laundry room once, too, by putting rags with gasoline in the dryer, literally blowing off the door to the laundry room. Daddy was a destructive man, and it was always someone else's fault—usually Cap's.

Cap wasn't allowed to play outside, until he was 9 or 10, and he wasn't allowed to have friends in the house, either. His dad was drinking or had a woman over or acted violent, and people visiting might uncover their "secrets." One of the secrets was where they lived. Every 2 or 3 years, Cap's mother would find them. Mom would try to go to their school to see Cap and his brother, but his dad had already told the teachers and counselors that his mom was dangerous, violent, and forbidden to see the kids, despite the "joint custody" ordered by the court. Cap would see his mom for a few moments, and a few times, his mom and dad got back together for a few days, which was really weird, but it happened. Then, his dad would move them. Suddenly, even in the middle of the night, they would pack everything up, and move to another city, to keep Cap from his mom.

Daddy was in construction. They would always have transient men, men without homes, crashing on their couch, lying all over the place in sleeping bags, hanging out and partying, and drinking until all hours of the night. Cap hated them, and he was disgusted by men: they were loud, cussing, womanizing, and got piss-drunk, urinating on the beds and furniture, trashing the house Cap tried to keep clean.

When he was allowed to go play in the neighborhood, like other "normal" kids, Cap didn't like playing with the other boys. He rejected the typical boy play of rough and tumble, running around and fighting and yelling and playing sports. Cap didn't like all the "boys" stuff, that reminded him of his dad, and he didn't want to be like his dad. Cap liked hanging out with the girls: talking, sitting around in groups, playing quietly, laughing, cooking, and liking each other. At 10, Charles learned to bake. He read cookbooks and watched T.V., and learned to make a chocolate cake from scratch: 2 cups of flour, one cup of cocoa, butter, etc . . . He still remembers his first cooking accomplishment. Daddy didn't like that. Daddy called him names, "wimp, sissy" and worse.

Cap's little brother, Damon, the spitting image of his father, turned out just dad. Even as a little boy, his brother was very, very mean. And Daddy would let Damon get away with it, treating Cap that way, always taking Damon's side. Everything was always Cap's fault. When they became teenagers, Damon started growing weed in their backyard, and got his hand on guns to protect him from bad boys. Cap told his dad about it, but his dad looked the other way and wouldn't deal with it.

When Cap was 12, his dad remarried and he got a stepmother, with whom he got along pretty well. His stepmother started teaching him survival skills. Even at 14, she helped him write up flyers, the kind with strips of paper and phone numbers on the bottom you see in grocery stores, to get jobs cleaning apartments and babysitting. She taught him about making money and saving money, and buying his own clothes and personal items. Money gave him freedom: to wear the clothes he wanted, to express himself, and gave him a sense of individual power.

Cap says that "Everything I know, I know from women." His stepmother, and other women, taught him to cook, shop, and most importantly, talk to girls, and how to treat girls. Girls taught him how to laugh, like, love, and connect to people. Girls and women were the one survival tool in his life. They taught him how to feel, listen, respond to people and emotions, and they taught him how to treat girls, too. Women were the one blessing in his life.

By 16, Cap was disgusted with his home life, his brother's drug dealing, and he left home. He dropped out of high school, got his GED, and went to vocational training. In a year, he finished a certificate that could get him a job. Cap spent a year, while he was in school, living on a couch in a single wide trailer that was old and had holes in the floor, not to mention cockroaches and mice, with a young married couple that fought all the time. But, he finished school and began living independently on his own at the age of 17.

Cap's message to boys is: Be aware and considerate of other people's feelings. First, start with truth!

What Every Guy Needs to Know About Physical and Sexual Abuse

Cap, a broken boy, was rescued by his connections to girls and women. As he said, "Women were the one blessing in his life." Cap lived a young life exposed to violence from his father, and he rejected his role model of "manhood." Being a man meant to be a womanizer, an abuser, a liar, a cheat, and hurting other people, especially women. Fortunately, Cap became friends with girls and close with women. He learned to talk, listen, nurture, work, laugh, and even cook! Everything he learned, he learned from women. Women were gentler, loving, and accepting. From women, he learned to treat girls right. As a result, he was very successful with women, even from a young age, around 13 and 14. He always had girlfriends and friends that were girls. Even though he was exposed to a great deal of violence, he took a different path, and he learned to have very loving relationships with people.

Cap's brother, Damon, became exactly opposite of Cap. He was mean as a child, and mean as a teenager. He was mean to his brother, then mean to his girlfriends, and became physically violent with them, just like his dad did to his mom. Often, boys who grow up watching or experiencing physical violence also become physically violent in their relationships with girls, as early as in their teenage years, when in dating relationships. The violence usually starts in a very small way, with verbal criticism and belittling, then increases to physical violence.

Cap's story, completely true, is a bad case scenario of how men can treat women, and how men treat boys, and how not to be a man in this world. Yet, many boys experience even a small parts of what Cap experienced growing up.

Boys who grow up with emotional and physical abuse, like Cap and his brother Damon, can either become abusers, like their parents, or try to do exactly the opposite of their parents, like Cap. Becoming an abuser is often a learned bad habit. It is what people do when they get stressed out. Sadly, often it doesn't work to solve problems and the abuse can escalate or increase over time. In the section below, types of abuse increase in the level of violence from emotional to physical violence.

Dating Violence: From Emotional to Physical Abuse

Emotional

- Criticism
- Insults
- Accusations
- Possessiveness
- Harsh demands
- Yelling
- Cursing
- Threats

Physical

- Pushing
- Grabbing a hand
- Grabbing a wrist
- Grabbing both upper arms
- Shoving
- Slapping
- Punching
- Kicking
- Shaking
- Burning

Sexual

- Fondling
- Grabbing or grobing

- Exposing oneself
- Mastubating in front of someone w/o permission
- Sexual Touch without permission
- Any sexual penetration
- Date rape: oral, vaginal, anal

The Pattern of Abuse

Abuse Escalates

Often, abuse escalates, which means it starts out small, then it grows and increases over time. Often, abuse starts with emotional abuse, with criticism, which most people experience within their families or with their friends. Frankly, it is part of a parent's job to tell you when you are doing something wrong, and if you have a good friend, they will tell you the truth and tell you when you're messing up. So, some criticism is a normal part of life. Yet, criticism can go overboard, and the line is often reached when you received downright insults. For example, your girlfriend might say to you, "Hey, you really should have studied more for that test!" when she knows you were blowing off studying and playing video games all night long. On the other hand, if she says, "You're a total loser and you're never going to amount to anything in your life!" That is an insult! If you find yourself giving or receiving insults on a regular basis, take a step back, and evaluate your relationship. Sure, people have bad days and make mistakes once in a while, but if the insults escalate to worse behavior and more frequent worse behavior, you may be in an abusive relationship. Or if you're the one saying it, you may be an abuser. Also, being negative and critical all the time can be a sign of depression. If someone is normally a nice person, then seems irritable and angry all the time, and it's not just hormonal for a couple of days, think twice about depression.

Blaming Others

Another classic part of the abuse is that abusers blame their victim. No matter what happens, the victim gets blamed. Like in Cap's story: when his father blew up the laundry room by putting gasoline soaked rags in the dryer, it was Cap's fault, because he was supposed to do the laundry. Abusers have a very hard time accepting responsibility for their actions. They twist everything around and make it someone else's fault. They have a very hard time saying they are wrong and then saying they are sorry. Not being able to admit fault also makes it very hard to solve any problem, because they don't think they need to change! They are never wrong! Are you ever wrong? Can YOU say you're sorry?

269

Broken Boys: Rage and Pity

A lot of abusers are also broken boys. Many broken boys have been abused and they are scared deep inside. The fear leaves them with two emotions: rage and pity. The rage is what you see with abuse. The pity is what you see when the abuser is about to lose everything. When Cap's dad's house burned down, he broke down in sobs, "I'm going to lose everything!" Sob, sob, sob! Cap's mom came back, feeling sorry for Cap's dad. His dad said, "I'm so sorry for everything. I was wrong about everything. I'll change everything. I'll never hit you again. I love you so much." Teenage guys will do this, too, with their girlfriend, who has been insulted or pushed or yelled at and is going to break up with them. At first, they'll act like they don't care, "I didn't do anything wrong, get over it!" Then, when they're afraid they'll lose her for good, they'll call and put on the big pity act, "I'm so sorry, you're right! Everything you said was right! I was wrong! I'll never do it again! I'll DO ANYTHING!" It works, she takes him back.

Honeymoon Phase

The next part of the abuse cycle is the honeymoon phase. For a little while, things are really good, very good. Usually, the guy acts really, really nice. He is the perfect boyfriend. He says everything every girl ever wants to hear. He buys her a really nice present, like a new cell phone, something way over the top, or the birthday present he "forgot" to give her, he goes overboard, and she really thinks he loves her. He proves it. Heck, Cap's dad bought his mom a new, used trailer! That is love!

The honeymoon might last a week, two weeks, or a couple of months, but it doesn't last. Yet, during this time, love seems so perfect, that couples seem to get addicted to this perfect "romantic love." The rage returns, because the normal human emotions of compassion, and a sense of responsibility are not there or in teenage guys, may not be developed with maturity, yet. A lot of time abuse happens because guys may be inexperienced problem solvers, they get frustrated and don't know how to deal, so they just get angry. Girls can have these problems, too. Once the honeymoon phase is over, the abuse starts again, only it escalates: it gets worse.

Physical abuse in teen relationships is a very serious problem affecting millions of teens a year. Forty percent of teens say they know someone who is in a violent relationship and one in three teens will experience a violent relationship. The only way to end the violence is to end the relationship. Period. Often, girls and guys will go back and forth in a relationship, going through a cycle of abuse, a break-up, a honeymoon phase, a cycle of abuse, a break-up, a honeymoon phase, and so on, several times, until someone gets hurt. If you know someone who is in a violent relationship, you need to talk to them and try to explain to them what is going on, and let them read this chapter. The problem won't go away, it will more than likely be repeated in future relationships and they need professional help.

If you have been emotionally or physically abused, or if you have found yourself being abusive, you need to seek professional help. A list of National Hotline phone numbers are at the end of this chapter. A good place to start is 1–800–4-CHILD. Most counties have professional mental health associations.

COMMON TYPES OF SEXUAL ABUSE

One in seven boys is sexually molested or abused by the time he reaches the age of 18. It happens to boys, too. Sexual silence, guilt, and embarrassment prevent boys from talking about sexual abuse. Fear of exposing a family member or family friend to criminal prosecution and disrupting one's family or extended family is another very real reason boys, even more often than girls, keep silent about sexual abuse. Often abuse happens in the context of a trusted relationship, even though the victim himself is betrayed, and it may involve threats of physical harm if he tells. Fear and guilt breed silence.

Sexual abuse can affect a boy in profound ways. Tragically, trusting people is one of the most difficult problems, even trusting talking to a counselor. Yet, seeking help as an teen is very important, since many young men have problems with depression, school, sleeping, nightmares, panic attacks, drugs and alcohol, and sex. As a teen, you can legally talk to a counselor confidentially, without them telling anything to your parents. Counselors are required to report sexual abuse if it is currently ongoing and a minor is in danger, but counselors can not report an abuser if they do not know their name, that is, if the abuser's name is not revealed.

Wendy Maltz, an author and expert on sexual abuse, writes in *The Sexual Healing Journey* (1991, page 31): "Sexual abuse occurs whenever one person dominates and exploits another by means of sexual activity or suggestion.

Sexual feelings and behavior that are used to degrade, humiliate, control, hurt, or otherwise misuse another person are sexually abusive. Coercion or betrayal often plays into sexual abuse. The abuse can take a direct, painful, and obvious course, such as in stranger rape. Or abuse can be indirect, perhaps even subtle, such as when a victim is gently fondled by an offender who professes love."

TYPES OF SEXUAL ABUSE

Exhibitionism or exposure: Displaying the naked body or parts of the naked body in an effort to shock, intimidate, or sexually arouse a victim.

Molestation: Sexual abuse involving sexual stimulation to body and genital areas, usually by touch, but also including penis to vagina or anus or mouth. It can happen at any age and by a perpetrator of any age.

Child sexual abuse: Sexual abuse of children by adults or by older children or peers who dominate and control through sexual activity. Older boys may make younger boys undress and then touch them genitally, for example. Childhood sexual abuse can be committed by a stranger, but most often it is done by adults or older children in trusted caretaking roles. A rule of thumb for "normal sexual exploration" by children with children is an age difference of no more than 3 years, and includes undressing, nudity, hugging and kissing, but not sexual touch.

Incest: Incest is the most common form of child sexual abuse. Incest is sexual abuse of children by other family members, including mothers or fathers, sisters and brothers, stepparents, aunts, uncles, cousins, and grandparents.

Date or acquaintance rape: Sexual abuse and sexual behavior for which there is no verbal or nonverbal permission. This type of rape may be sexual assault, but it is not necessarily violent. Date rape is committed by someone known to the victim, often a peer in a trusted social relationship.

Stranger rape: Violence, anger, and power expressed sexually in an attack on a victim. It may involve penetration of body openings (mouth, anus, vagina), but it does not have to. Stranger rape is a sexual attack committed by someone unknown to the victim.

Marital rape: Rape of a spouse or marital partner. Yes, you must have permission to have sex with your wife or husband.

Sexual assault: A physical attack to a victim's sexual body parts, often involving force or violence. This term can cover a wide rage of activities and can include the rape of boys and men.

Voyeurism: An invasion of a victim's privacy either secretively or openly with the intent of gaining sexual gratification. Commonly, this can mean watching someone having sexual relations, watching someone dress, or just watching someone for sexual gratification, such as a man in a truck stalking a girl in a car while she is riding down the highway with a short skirt on. This person can also be called a "peeping Tom."

Obscene phone calls: An invasion of a victim's privacy with sexually suggestive messages over the telephone in an effort to shock, intimidate, or sexually arouse a victim. Often the offender will be doing this for sexual excitement and may be masturbating.

Statutory rape: If you are younger than a certain age, having sex is child sexual abuse, even if you say "yes." If you are younger than the age of consent, anyone having sex with you is committing statutory rape. "Statutory" means it is a crime because of your status, the status in this case being a minor who is not the age of consent. The age of consent is how old a child must be to legally say it is OK to have sexual touch or sexual intercourse, or else it is legally considered sexual assault or molestation or rape. The idea is that young people could be coerced into sex, which means that they are not yet ready to make this decision based on their age. See Chapter Four on "The Legal Bottom Line" on sex.

What Every Guy Needs to Know About Physical and Sexual Abuse

Sadistic sexual abuse: Sadistic means cruel or vicious. Sexual abuse in which the offender incites or tries to incite reactions of dread, horror, or pain in the victim, often increasing the offender's sexual arousal during the abuse, is sadistic sexual abuse. This may involve use of physical restraint, religious types of rituals, multiple perpetrators, animals, and torture.

Sexual exploitation: Using a person as a thing, not as a real person, or "objectifying" a victim in sexual activity or photographic imagery to gain money for sexual gratification.

Sexual harassment: Generally, sexual harassment happens in a school or workplace, where a person uses his or her power or status to intimidate or control a victim, perhaps requiring sexual involvement. One type of sexual harassment may be expressed as excessive sexual flirtatiousness, and/or requests for sexual favors to obtain something from the abused, such as undressing or having sex for a good grade in a class. The other type of sexual harassment involves creating a "sexually hostile" environment, such as continually making degrading comments about women, displaying explicit sexual pictures, or telling dirty sex jokes.

Gender attack: An exposure to actions that demean the sexual gender of a victim, often with sexual overtones, such as cross-dressing a child or verbally denigrating a victim's gender.

Gay bashing: Verbal or physical attacks directed against a victim's perceived homosexual orientation.

Sexual violence: Acts of violence involving or harming or violating the sexual parts of the victim's body.

THE INTERNET: A CAUTIONARY TALE

Instant messaging on the Internet is the most popular way for teens to socialize. In the 50s it was the "soda shop," where our grandparents went to drink cherry cokes and hang out with friends. In the 70s, it was the telephone. Having your own "teen phone," to talk on for 2 or 3 hours a day was the way 14 year olds "got together." Now, teens use the Internet and chat online, whether it's AOL or AIM, to socialize.

Teens can talk to teens from their local hometown to Singapore to anywhere in the world on the Internet. As many as 80% of teens are online, with many of them using instant messaging to reach out to friends or get to know new friends they might meet in chatrooms. Instant messaging or "IMing" as a way to socialize is a fun, quick, and easy way to stay in touch. Having four screens going at a time and typing quickly is a way to keep your social life moving fast. Most of the time, it is a safe and fun way to "get together." Yet, the amazing statistic is that 15% (FIFTEEN percent) of teens actually meet people they meet online LIVE and in person. Often these meetings are private, secretive, without parental knowledge or consent, with teens meeting strangers they have only met online.

Kids are taught, "Don't talk to strangers," from the time they can understand language. Yet, as teens, millions of people are meeting strangers everyday on the Internet, and thousands of teens are meeting strangers in person every year. Strange, isn't it? You know not to talk to strangers, yet, it has become commonplace to talk to people you don't really know online every day! Making the leap from the anonymous contact of the world wide web and Internet chatting to meeting a person live seems very different than the warnings we were taught as children, to stay away from strangers. After "talking" or chatting online, in a very short period of time, people can begin to feel very close, and experience feelings as deeply as if they were meeting in person. So, the leap from anonymous to meeting what seems to be a new, very best friend, doesn't seem like it is in the same category of meeting a stranger. Yet, in fact, you are meeting a stranger and it is very dangerous!

Meeting a stranger you have "met" online is very dangerous.

People can pretend to be anyone they want to be online. A 50-year-old, hairy, wrinkled older man, who is attracted to children, can pretend to be hot 16-year-old girl (or guy), who loves the same music as you do. Child sexual predators used teenage chatrooms to get individual email addresses, then use instant messaging to develop "relationships," then they prey on teens like an animal preys on another animal. Many teenagers have met people in person people they have met online: some of them have been sexually assaulted and even murdered. Teenagers are at great risk for becoming victims of child abuse, pornography, or even human trafficking (prostitution), when they meet strangers they have met online on the Internet.

Dos and Don'ts of the Internet

- Do not use an Internet name that has personal information, such as the name of your high school, town, or sport, e.g. "WashingtonHighFootball8."
- Never give out your phone number.
- Never give out your home town or address information.
- Do not tell your real name, especially your last name. Always use a nickname that your real friends already know.
- If you begin to feel uncomfortable when talking and meeting people online, leave the site and turn off your computer immediately.

- Do tell someone if someone starts asking really personal or inappropriate and/or sexual questions. If someone starts asking you a lot of personal questions, report them to https://web.cybertip.org/cyberTipII.html.

- Do not meet anyone you meet online.

- If you feel you must meet someone, always tell a parent, meet in a public place, and go with someone while having your own transportation to come and leave.

- Remember that if you call someone, they can get your phone number from their cell phone or they can get call *69 to get your number. If you ever make a phone call, don't call a cell phone number, or dial *67 first to block your phone number. If someone has your phone number, they can get your home address!

- A legitimate (for real) person will have no problems of your parents and/or friends knowing you are meeting them.

SEXUAL MOLESTATION

Charlie C's Story

We met Charlie C. in Chapter One, with his story of "the Knight in Shining Armor Syndrome," about his first sexual experience with a girl at 15. You might remember, when he was 13 and 14, he had a lot of girlfriends that he would kiss and hug and make-out. The girl, Jackie, asked Charlie to have sex with her. Charlie was worried it wasn't right. He wanted to be sensitive and understanding and he didn't want to pressure her or push her for sex. He didn't want her to feel like she "had to" do it. Really, he wanted to make sure it was really O.K. and he didn't want her to regret it. He thought a lot about her feelings and the "big picture," and how having sex with him might "change her." For a guy, Charlie was very sensitive to Jackie's thoughts, feelings, and desires. Charlie had his reasons.

When Charlie was a young boy, he was sexually molested and abused, by friends of his parents who were babysitting him.

Charlie was around six years old. Two guys were watching him, who were kind of young, maybe in their 20's, and friends of his parents. His parents had no idea that these men were sexual offenders. The first sign of something wrong was that they wanted to watch him going to the bathroom: they came in the bathroom, both of them and watched him pee. Charlie thought that was uncomfortable. Then, when he went to take a nap, they got into bed with him. They fondled his genitals. He didn't like it. He felt violated and upset.

Then an extremely strange thing happened. One day, one of the guys was in the kitchen with Charlie. He unzipped his pants, and masturbated and ejaculated right in front of him.

Charlie ran, as fast as he could run, to the next door neighbor's house, where an old black woman lived. When she opened the door, Charlie ran in and hid in her bathroom, behind a huge, claw foot bathtub. He stayed there and wouldn't come out until his parent's came over and found him and brought him home. He told his parents what had happened, as best as he could describe. Poor Charlie was shaking like a leaf in the corner of that bathroom, when they found him.

Maybe because of that, Charlie became very sensitive about never imposing himself on anyone, anywhere, anyway. He thought about how frightened he had been and he never wanted to make anyone feel that way. He never wanted to violate or hurt anyone. And, he never did.

Charlie was told from when he could remember, "If anyone touches your private parts, RUN!" Well, he ran! And, he told. Fortunately, he was protected by a neighbor, who was kind and caring, and even though he'd never even met her, she took care of him for hours. Charlie's parents were horrified, but they responded quickly and immediately and protected him. Sometimes, parents simply can't protect you from every possible danger, but they can help you from future danger, if you will let them. Even though they were family friends, his parents turned them into the police, and Charlie had to talk to about 15 different social workers and a judge before it was all over.

The one good thing that came out of the situation was that it made Charlie very sensitive to other people's sexual feelings. He remembers how frightened he was and he never wanted to hurt anyone. He didn't.

Sexual Abuse—South's Story

South was 8 years old when he first remembers being sexually abused by his uncle, his mother's brother. In the summers, South would spend the time on his grandparent's farm, since his mother was working, his Dad was long gone, and his mom thought it would be good for him to live in the country all summer long. Uncle Jay lived on the family farm at the time; he was 22. Uncle Jay was a reckless man. He partied and drove drunk, and didn't care about anyone else but himself.

Jay was a train wreck to everyone he met in his life. South's grandparents had six kids. Five of them went zig, Jay went zag.

Jay started abusing South when he was still in elementary school. Jay would make South perform oral sex on him, and gave him special favors for doing it. He would take him out for ice cream, which was a big treat for a poor country kid with no mom and dad around. South hated his Uncle. Jay tried to have anal sex with him, but South managed to run away. South was a little boy, who was physically and emotionally traumatized by the sexual abuse. He began to hide away from everyone on the farm, staying as far away from Jay as possible.

Confusion seemed to be the overwhelming word that occupied South's mind. Why was this happening to him and no one else? Did this mean that he was really gay or something? Then came the anger and the feelings of rage that there was no one to help him and no one to save him. South stopped playing sports because he was afraid that another kid would hit him or run into him and he would go into a rage and hurt them and maybe even kill them. With each passing day he became more quiet and withdrawn until something happened that he thought would release him from his hell. Uncle Jay was killed in an auto accident.

This great day of liberation was not allowed to be the release that he had hoped it would be. Uncle Jay did not do the world a favor and just kill himself; instead he was drunk and tried passing another car on a hill at night. An oncoming car with a family of 4 inside became his latest victims. Somehow South felt a great sadness for that family and connected to them because they were all victims of Jay. South never cried at Uncle Jay's funeral, except for the family he killed. He just prayed that family would all go to heaven together, as they all had died together. South wished he could die and go to heaven with the family, too. Somehow, he always felt a bond with them.

When South was a teenager, 15, he was told to go live with his cousin, Johnny, in the big city nearby. His mom thought it might be an opportunity for him to get a good education and to have the advantages that poverty in the country would never provide. The only condition was that South would live with his 27-year-old cousin and help around the house. Johnny was very attentive and showed South every part of St. Louis. At first, South had a lot of fun, riding the trolleys and being independent. After several weeks, his cousin started coming into his bedroom at night and began crawling into bed with South. The condition for living with his cousin included regular nightly sex, including anal sex, which was very painful, and at times sharing South with some of Johnny's closest friends. Johnny realized that

South had very strong sexual feelings for girls, so in order to keep South satisfied and remain with him in the city, a maid was hired to help around the house and take care of South, in every way.

South felt oh so trapped, but he felt he could do nothing to get out of his situation with his cousin. He did not feel he could tell his mother and go home. His mom was an alcoholic and barely managed taking care of his brother and sister. South felt that she already couldn't manage the pain in her life. He didn't want to send his mom over the edge by telling her that he was being sexually abused by a family member, and put her and the family into a state of turmoil. South was a sensitive boy and he tried to protect his mother, by allowing the abuse to continue. He felt he was stronger than his mom and he could take the abuse more than she could take the trauma. He sacrificed himself for his family, or at least that is what he thought was the best thing at the time.

One day South had what he always thought was a message from God. One night when South was in bed, frightfully waiting for Johnny to come into his bedroom, he felt the presence of God inside himself. He heard the words, "Run, get away, leave at all costs, leave now!" South suddenly left the city and returned home. South never said a word to anyone about what had happened. His cousin never called him or tried to come after him. Johnny died several years later of AIDS. South was thrilled, once again, with the death of his abuser.

Finally freed after Johnny's death, and after a first failed marriage, wondering what was wrong with him, South entered therapy for the first time. Then, he began a journey of healing and living, not just surviving.

South never told anyone about his sexual abuse until after his divorce, when he went into therapy. He felt too ashamed to admit that a man had sex with him. He was afraid that someone, even a therapist, but certainly a girlfriend or wife, would think he was gay, or that it was his fault. Why didn't he leave sooner? Why didn't he tell his grandparents? He was ashamed to talk about sex, let alone say that someone was having sex with him. He didn't want to get his uncle, nor his cousin sent to jail and break his grandmother's heart or his aunt's or his mother's. He felt that, as a young man, he was strong enough to handle the pain of sexual abuse, more than they could handle the pain of having someone in their family go to jail. South also didn't know if anyone would believe him: a kid! And, he was afraid everyone would be mad at him! When you're a kid, you're afraid that when something bad happens, it's your fault, even when it's not, and often boys take the blame.

Therapy saved South's life. Like a lot of sexual abuse survivors, South didn't think he'd live to 18, or to 30. He went through a lot of depression. And a failed marriage. Today, after a few years of therapy, South is happily married.

> South's message to boys is: Tell. I told my mother when I was 30 years old. She was so sad that I felt I couldn't tell her as a child. She wished she could have been there for me, no matter what was happening in her life. She knew her brother was bad, but not that bad. She wished she could have protected me, but my silence never gave her a chance. I am sure now that she would have done everything she could have to take care of me, and it would have saved me a lot of pain.

What To Do If You Are Sexually Assaulted

1. Go to a friend or a family member. Do not be alone!

2. If one person does not believe you or want to be with you,

try another, then another, then another, if necessary. Or call
a National Hotline 1–800–656-HOPE.

3. Get medical attention. Tell them you were raped and make
   sure they use a rape kit.

4. Report the rape to the police.

5. Get professional counseling starting immediately.

6. Do not blame yourself . . . no matter what.

7. Remember: It happens to boys, too. It's just not *you.*

DATE RAPE

Acquaintance and Date Rape

"Date rape" is forced, unwanted sex with someone the victim is dating. Acquaintance rape is forced, unwanted sexual intercourse by
a person the victim knows. Date rape is the term commonly used
for the sexual assault of a woman by a man. Boys are vulnerable to
date raped, too, especially gay males, but it is less common. Guys are
vulnerable to acquaintance rape in college, from fraternity hazings
and parties. More commonly, date rape is when a guy forces sexual
relations on a girl, although many times, guys and even some girls,
do not call it rape.

Rape Statistics

- A girl is raped every 2 minutes in the United States.
- 9% of rapes are of males
- 28% of girls are raped by their boyfriends
- 35% of women are raped by acquaintances
- 5% are raped by relatives

- Less than one third of rapes are reported, and up to 90% of college date rapes are not reported
- 44% of rape victims are under 18.
- 90% of date rapes happen when the victim or attacker is drinking or using drugs
- 25% of college women are victims of date rape
- 8.9% of college men admit date rape—but don't consider it rape
- 50–75% of college women, initially, don't consider date rape as rape
- 33% of men said they would date rape someone if it could go undetected
- 44% of women who were date raped have considered suicide.

(http://womenissues.about.com/od/rapecrisis/a/rapestats.htm)

Most startling among the statistics are how common rape is, that it happens every two minutes, and that one in four girls in college is raped. One of every four girls that you know now in high school or college, your friend, your sister, you're your cousin, your mother, your aunt, your teacher, has been or will be raped. The chances are very high that they know who raped them, up to 84% of the time. Amazingly, one third of college aged men said that they would commit date rape, if they could get away with it, while 44% of women who went through the trauma were so horribly affected by it, they wanted to commit suicide and die! Often, girls blame themselves, most likely because they knew the rapist, they question what really happened, they were often drinking and blamed themselves

284

for "leading someone on," or putting themselves in a bad situation, which is why, initially, some girls don't consider date rape, rape.

While some guys might not think of forced sex as rape, this action is a serious crime—a felony. Whenever a man uses force to have sex, even when he knows the woman, even when they have had sex before, even if they are married or engaged, even if you are just about to have sex and she says no, even if you're naked and making out and she changed her mind, it is a crime.

> If convicted of Date Rape, your name is placed for the rest of your life on the National Sex Offender Registry, which is listed on the Internet, in addition to serving a criminal sentence for rape.

What Guys Need to Know to Prevent Date Rape

- Don't make assumptions that because a girl wants to have other sexual touch, such as oral sex, that she also wants sexual intercourse.
- Don't assume that if she's had sex with you before, it's OK to have sex again.
- Don't assume that a girl wants to have sex with you, just because she's flirting with you or she goes to a room alone with you, or she's "dressed for sex."
- Don't assume that you're "entitled" to have sex just because you've spent a lot of money on a date.
- Do listen closely to what a girl is saying. If she is not being direct, or the speech is muffled, take a second to make sure she is saying "yes," not "no," or "stop." Saying you thought you heard yes later is no defense for rape.
- Don't fall for the line that when a woman says "no," she really means "yes," or "maybe," or "convince me." If a woman says "no," stop. Believe me, if she says yes, you'll hear it, loud and clear.

- Don't have sex with someone who is mentally or physically incapable of giving consent to sex. If you have sex with a women who is heavily intoxicated, passed out, drugged, or incapable of saying "yes," OR "no," you may be guilty of rape.
- Don't participate in group situations, with a group of guys having sex with a girl, when the guy says the girl said it's OK to have sex with her. Walk away from these situations, or better yet, get the girl out of there or get help for her!
- Do get involved if you see a girl in trouble. If you see a guy pressuring a girl, or someone really drunk and passing out and leaving with a guy, don't be afraid to intervene! You may save that girl from the trauma of rape or being killed, and your friend from the ordeal of criminal prosecution.
- Don't coerce a girl into having sex. If you make threats to force a girl to have sex with you, it's rape. For example, if you tell her that if she doesn't have sex with you, you'll tell her parents and all her friends and her boyfriend that you had sex anyway, unless she has sex with you right then, that is emotional coercion. Emotional coercion for sex can be considered rape, too.
- Do not use force to have sex with someone. If you are using any kind of force, whether you are holding someone down, refusing to leave their room or apartment, or using a weapon, this is rape. The victim might not actually say, "NO," because she is afraid for her LIFE, and very frightened, but the use of force is coerced sex and rape.

All rape is traumatic, but there is something particularly traumatic about a man or woman being raped by someone they know and had previously liked and trusted. It can make a person stop trusting all people and the whole world, at least for a while. For some, the lack of trust and dislike of people can last for many years.

False Accusations of Rape

People do lie about rape or sexual assault. The Kobe Bryant case may be a recent example of false accusation. Estimates of false accusations vary widely, but at least 10% of the time, "victims" lie, and up to 50% of the time, research has found accusations to be false. Women (and men) lie because of spite, a desire for revenge, a need for an alibi, and feelings of guilt or shame later. Yet, because rape is such an emotionally charged issue, and a crime, the accusation of rape can get a young man into very serious trouble. One accusation of rape will turn a person's life completely upside down and cost him everything — his job, his family, his home, money, and respect. One of the problems with false accusations is that often a guy is often seen as guilty until proven innocent. Usually, no one believes the person, and once accused, living down the reputation can take a very long time, if not the rest of his life.

False accusations can be also be made in child sexual assault cases, although it has only been proven to happen less than 10% of the time. While that is a relatively smaller number, for the innocent person who is accused and presumed guilty, such a situation will have devastating effects on their life.

287

Your Sexual Rights

The right to develop healthy attitudes about sex

The right to sexual privacy

The right to protect yourself from bodily invasion and harm

The right to say no to sexual behavior

The right to control touch and sexual contact

The right to stop sexual excitement that feels inappropriate

The right to develop your sexuality according to your sexual
preferences and orientation

The right to enjoy healthy sexual pleasure and satisfaction

(Reprinted with the permission of Wendy Maltz, MSW, AASECT Certified
Sex Therapist)

288

nning pregnancy why say no planning why say 10 question quiz
onships how do I know when am I ready? plannir
ual voice to make the best personal choice oes he
ationships how to say no relationships love pregna
say no planning why say 10 question quiz dating pregnancy rela

VIRGIN SEX

www.noregretsguide.com

About the Website

If *Virgin Sex for Guys* got you wondering what other teens thought of these topics, come visit our companion website, www.noregretsguide.com. There, you can download and view video clips of your peers discussing everything in this book—and more!

Short video clips can be downloaded right to your computer. Find out what other teens thought about the "Are You Ready for Sex?" Quiz, religious values and sex, birth control, date rape, having (and not having) sex, coming out, relationship lies, and the other topics covered in *Virgin Sex for Guys*.

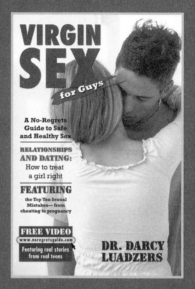

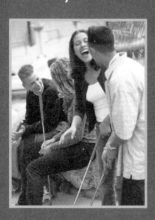

While you're there, take the time to ask Dr. Darcy your own sex question, read and comment on Dr. Darcy's blog, and browse the archive of frequently asked questions and other resources. You can stay completely anonymous. If this book has left something unanswered, please come and ask. Join the conversation, learn more about safe and healthy sex, download videos of teens in open debate, and much more—it's all part of the community of teens at www.noregretsguide.com.

s when am I ready? planning why say no no-regrets why we have
thoughts date rape avoiding situations that could how to develop
voice to make the best personal choice does he like you? protectio
shipshow to say norelationships love pregnancywhy say no plannii
10 question quiz dating pregnancy relationshipshow to know

Bibliography

Alanguttmacher.org. The Guttmacher Institute, New York and Washington, 2006.

Basso, Michael J. *The Underground Guide to Teenage Sexuality*. Fairview Press, 1997.

Bell, Ruth. *Changing Bodies, Changing Lives: A Book for Teens on Sex and Relationships*. Random House, 1998.

Dodson, Betty. *Sex for One: The Joy of Self Loving*. Random House, 1987.

Hughes, Jean, and Sandler, Bernice. *Friends Raping Friends*. Association of American Colleges, 1987.

Maltz, Wendy. *The Sexual Healing Journey*. HarperCollins Publishers, 1991.

Masters, W., Johnson, V. Human Sexual Response. Little, Brown, 1966.

Mosher, WD, Chandra, A, Jones, J. Sexual Behavior and selected health measures: Men and Women 15–44 years of age. United States, 2002. Advance data from vital and health statistics, no 367. Hyattsville, MD. National Center for Health Statistics, 2005.

Nakashima, AK, Rolfs, RT, Flock, ML, Kilmarx, P, Greenspan, JR. *Epidemiology of syphilis in the US 1941 through 1993*. Sexually Transmitted Diseases, 1196, 23:16–23.

National Child Exploitation Coordination Centre (NCECC). Internet Based Sexual Exploitation of Children and Youth Environmental Scan, http://ncecc.ca/enviroscan_2005_e.htm, 2005.

National Center for Missing and Exploited Children. "Don't Believe the Type," 2006.

Planned Parenthood. *The Emergency Contraception Handbook*. Planned Parenthood Federation of America, March, 1999.

290

Resource Listings

Free Telephone Hotline Numbers

Adolescent Crisis Intervention & counseling Nineline
1-800-999-9999

AIDS National Hotline
1-800-342-2437

Al-Anon/Alateen Hotline
1-800-344-2666

Alcohol/Drug Abuse Hotline
1–800–662-HELP

Be Sober Hotline
1–800-BE-SOBER

Child Abuse Hotline
1–800–4-A-CHILD

Cocaine Hotline
1–800-Cocaine

Domestic Violence Hotline
1-800-548-2722

Emergency Contraception Information
1–800-NOT-2-LATE

Family Violence
1-800-313-1310

Gay & Lesbian National Hotline
  1–888-THE-GLNH (843-4564)

Gay, Lesbian, Bisexual, and Trangender (GLBT) Youth Support Line
  1-800-850-8078

Help Finding a Therapist
  1–800-THERAPIST

Homeless/Runaway National Hotline
  1-800-231-6946

Incest Hotline for guys: M.A.L.E.
  1–800–949-MALE

National Adolescent Suicide Hotline
  1-800-621-4000

National Association for Children of Alcoholics
  1–800–55-4CHOAS (1-888-554-2627)

National Abortion Federation Hotline
  1-800-772-9100

National Adoption Center
  1-800-648-4400

National Child Abuse Hotline
  1-800-422-4453

National Drug Abuse Hotline
  1–800–622-HELP

National STD Hotline
  1-800-227-8922

National Youth Crisis Hotline
  1-800-448-4663

National Victim Center
  1–800-FYI-CALL

People Against Rape
1-800-877-7252

Planned Parenthood
1–800–230-PLAN

Pregnancy Hotline
1–800–4-OPTIONS

Pregnant & Young Hotline (Birthright)
1-800-550-4900

Rape, Abuse, Incest, National Network (RAINN)
1–800–656-HOPE

Runaway Hotline
1-800-231-6946

Safe Choice Hotline (STDs & Pregnancy)
1-800-878-2347

Self-Injury Hotline
1–800-DON'T-CUT

Sexual Assault Hotline
1-800-656-4673

Stop it Now! (Sexual Abuse)
1–800-PREVENT

TalkZone (Peer Counselors—other teens)
1–800–475-TALK

TeenLine
1-800-522-8336

The Trevor HelpLine (specializing in gay and lesbian youth suicide prevention)
1-800-850-8078

Youth Crisis Hotline
    1-800-448-4663
    1-800-422-0009

WEBSITE LISTINGS/RESOURCES

Internet Dangers
    http://tcs.cybertipline.com/knowthedangers1.htm

Teenwire.com
    Planned parenthood site for sexual health information

DrDarcyonline.com
    Free online sex question and more info about Dr. Darcy

Index

295

C

can I handle having a relationship with a girl, including possible rejection?, 101–107

can we legally have sex, 128–132

casual sex, 171

cervical cap, 215–216

cheating, 52–53

Child Abuse Hotline, 290

child sexual abuse, 272

child support, 109

chlamydia, 190–191

clap, 197

clitoral hood, 181

clitoris, 163, 165, 181

cluelessness, 1

Cocaine Hotline, 290

comfortable with a girl, feeling, 225–226

coming out, 80–83

communication, importance of, 45–50

conditions for sex, 16, 17, 92–93

condoms, 124, 181, 215

continuous abstinence, 181

contraceptive foams, 217

contraceptive gels, 217

coyote ugly, 133

crabs, 198–199

crushes, 151–153

curiosity, 22–26

D

date rape, 272, 283–287

Depo-Provera, 217–218

development of sex, 135

diaphragm, 182, 215–216

dildo, 182

do I really know enough about how sex works, 98–101

Domestic Violence Hotline, 290

Dr. Darcy's "Am I Ready for Sex" Quiz, 90

Dr. Darcy's Guide on How To Treat A Girl Right, 44–45

Dr. Darcy's Secret Three Step Solution for Communication, 48

drip, 197

dry humping, 249

dry sex, 249

E

ejaculation, 140, 179–180, 182

emergency contraception, 219

Emergency Contraception Information, 290

emotional abuse, 267

emotional side of sex

    comfortable with a girl, feeling, 225–226

    emotional trust, 225–226

    girls and the emotional-sexual connection, 226–227

    jealousy, 224–225

    overview, 223–224

    secret of sexual communication, 227–228

emotional trust, 225–226

empathy, 97

erections, 151–153, 182

exhibition, 272

exposure, 272

expressions, sexual, 159–160

F

failure, birth control, 211

Family Violence, 290

fantasies, 167–168

female ejaculation, 179–180

fertility awareness methods, 220

first sexual feelings, 136–140

foreplay, 182, 238–239

free sex, 22

free touch zone, 164

friendships, importance of, 40

frottage, 249

fun, having, 53–54

297

National Adolescent Suicide Hotline, 291
National Adoption Center, 291
National Association for Children of Alcoholics, 291
National Child Abuse Hotline, 291
National Drug Abuse Hotline, 291
National STD Hotline, 291
National Victim Center, 291
National Youth Crisis Hotline, 291
natural family planning, 220
no method of birth control, 213
no pain-ever, 61, 62
Norplant, 217

O

obscene phone calls, 273
oral sex, 170–171, 181, 247–248
orgasm, 176–178
orgasms, 172–181, 257
outercourse, 182, 214

P

Parent test, 35–36
parents and sex, 34–37
parents, meeting the, 58–59
penis, 166
People Against Rape, 292
perfect use, 212
periodic abstinence, 181, 213
periods. See menstruation
physical and sexual abuse, 260–261, 261–271
physical side of sex
    if a girl says "no," stop, 233
    no pain-ever, 233
    permission, 232–234
    three rules of sex, 232
Planned Parenthood, 292
porn and sex, 30–32
pornography, 142–146
Pregnancy Hotline, 292
pregnancy, unexpected, 108–121. See

also birth control and pregnancy
Pregnant & Young Hotline (Birthright), 292
premature ejaculation, 179
public lice, 198–199
pulling out, 218–219
pure virgin sex, 221–223

R

Rape, Abuse, Incest, National Network (RAINN), 292
ready for sex, how do I know when I am
    am I certain I am not pressuring or coercing someone into sex, 96–98
    am I comfortable enough with my girlfriend to talk about sex, 126–128
    am I not pressured to have sex by anyone, including myself, 93–95
    am I ready to use birth control and practice safer sex, 121–125
    can I handle having a relationship with a girl, including possible rejection?, 101–107
    can we legally have sex, 128–132
    conditions for sex, 92–93
    do I really know enough about how sex works, 98–101
    Dr. Darcy's "Am I Ready for Sex" Quiz, 90
    have I considered what would happen if she got pregnant, 108–121
    overview, 89
    top ten sexual mistakes guys make, 90–91
    would I have sex if I weren't drunk or high?, 132–135
relationships, 40
relaxation, 180
religion and sex, 26–29

299

301